Student Workbook for

THE ADMINISTRATIVE
DENTAL ASSISTANT

Student Workbook for

THE ADMINISTRATIVE DENTAL ASSISTANT

Sixth Edition

Linda J. Gaylor, RDA, BPA, MEd
Retired Coordinator, Curriculum and Instruction
San Bernardino County Superintendent of Schools
Regional Occupational Program, Career Training, and Support Services
San Bernardino, California

ELSEVIER

Elsevier
3251 Riverport Lane
St. Louis, Missouri 63043

STUDENT WORKBOOK FOR THE ADMINISTRATIVE DENTAL ASSISTANT,
SIXTH EDITION

ISBN: 978-0-323-93609-5

Notice

Practitioners and researchers must always rely on their own experience and knowledge in evaluating and using any information, methods, compounds or experiments described herein. Because of rapid advances in the medical sciences, in particular, independent verification of diagnoses and drug dosages should be made. To the fullest extent of the law, no responsibility is assumed by Elsevier, authors, editors or contributors for any injury and/or damage to persons or property as a matter of products liability, negligence or otherwise, or from any use or operation of any methods, products, instructions, or ideas contained in the material herein.

Previous edition copyrighted 2021

Senior Content Strategist: Kelly Skelton
Senior Content Development Specialist: Rebecca Leenhouts
Publishing Services Manager: Deepthi Unni
Senior Project Manager: Kamatchi Madhavan
Design Direction: Gopal Venkatraman

Printed in India

Last digit is the print number: 9 8 7 6 5 4 3 2 1

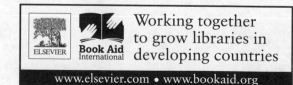

Introduction

TO THE STUDENT

The Student Workbook and Evolve companion website have been designed to help you perfect the skills and objectives presented in *The Administrative Dental Assistant*, sixth edition. To help you achieve these objectives, this workbook includes the following features:

- An **Introduction** briefly states the key concept and goals of each chapter.
- **Learning Objectives** identify the concepts and skills that are necessary to master the goal of each chapter.
- **Exercises** ask questions that require you to list information, identify key concepts, and match terms with their definitions. Short-answer questions direct you to solve problems and sequence activities. These exercises are intended to help you achieve the objectives in the textbook by providing a means by which you can study, work with others, and develop necessary skills.
- **Activity Exercises** help you apply information learned to complete tasks that are similar to tasks you will encounter as an administrative dental assistant. The activities require you to use information assembled in one activity to complete the next task. It is very important that you complete the tasks in the order in which they are presented. Before moving on to the next task, you should verify the correctness of the completed task. Referring to information identified in the "Anatomy of…" figures and procedures outlined in the textbook may prove helpful. *Remember:* The tasks are sequenced and must be completed in the order presented.
- **Dentrix Learning Edition Lessons** are assignments that you will complete online. The lessons provide how-to videos and exercises for you to practice working in Dentrix.
- **Dentrix Application Exercises** introduce you to a *real-world* dental practice management software and are designed to help develop basic skills. Dentrix is a leader in dental practice management software and dental office technology integration. The Evolve Resources website for the *Administrative Dental Assistant* text now has the Dentrix Learning Edition, a special version of Dentrix G7 designed specifically for educational purposes. It includes a preloaded database of patients and is interactive, allowing you to perform various tasks the way they are done in a dental office. The accompanying *User's Guide* walks you through all the tasks and functions of the program and provides an opportunity for you to explore more advanced functions of the dental practice management software.
- **Dentrix Learning Outcomes** will clearly state what you will be able to do when all of the assignments have been successfully completed.
- **The Dentrix User's Guide Resources** will direct you to sections of the User's Guide that will provide detailed information and instruction on the use of the software.
- **Dentrix Guided Practice** is a series of tasks that will guide you through step by step, so you become familiar with the software. During the guided practice you may have student assignment that will ask you questions or instruct you to use specific information, these are designed to help you apply certain knowledge and skills.
- **Dentrix Independent Practice** exercises will give you the opportunity to apply what you have learned to tasks that will be expected of an administrative assistant.
- **Dental Practice Procedural Manual Project** is an optional project that provides a way for you to *practice* various Career Ready Practices, such as collaboration, teamwork, critical thinking, communications, and application of technical skills. By working on this project, which spans the full textbook, your team will do research, have discussions, and come to consensus about the information you will include in your procedural manual. The majority of the information your team will need will be in the textbook and created during the Career Ready Practices exercises at the end of each chapter.
- The companion Evolve Resources website for *The Administrative Dental Assistant* was created specifically to help enhance the experiences of both students and instructors using the textbook and workbook. Accessible via http://evolve.elsevier.com/Gaylor/ada, the following resources are provided for students:
  - Dentrix Learning Edition Software
  - Computer Application Exercises
  - Dentrix Learning Edition Lesson Assignments
  - Interactive Forms
  - Practice Quizzes

Plus...

"Day in the Life" Simulation Tool

The features of this interactive software are designed to guide you through simulated tasks typical to a dental business office. For each day of the week in the program, the level of difficulty is increased and new concepts are introduced. Concepts are directly related to material in the textbook. On later days of the week you will be required to independently apply information and concepts that you have learned in the textbook. You may find the exercises to have more significance after completing Chapters 3 through 17.

The interactive program simulates a "Day in the Life of an Administrative Dental Assistant" and challenges you to complete tasks as they would occur in the workplace, such as organizing functions, prioritizing tasks, solving problems, and completing daily tasks typical of an administrative dental assistant. Exam and study modes incorporated into the program provide flexibility in teaching and learning. Whereas the exam mode requires you to log in and complete the tasks in order from Monday through Friday, tracking your progress and outputting a results sheet, the study mode allows you to enter any day and time throughout the weeklong exercise to practice or review specific procedures.

- A variety of tasks typical in practice management software are included: entering and updating patient data, posting payment and treatment procedures, submitting insurance e-claims for payment, evaluating reports, and scheduling appointments.
- Patients arrive for appointments, and you must complete related tasks such as updating patient information and completing the checkout process. The mail arrives on a daily basis and must be processed. The telephone rings, and you must take care of the caller.
- Pop-ups ask you questions about a particular subject relevant to the task at hand. Prompts indicate whether you have answered each question correctly or incorrectly and provide a rationale. (You can go back and view the correct response if you have answered incorrectly.)

I hope that you will find the textbook and the accompanying material useful in pursuing an exciting career as a member of a dental healthcare team.

Linda J. Gaylor

Contents

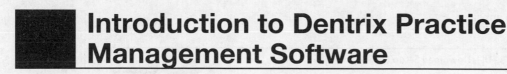

Introduction to Dentrix Practice Management Software

TIPS FOR A SUCCESSFUL INSTALLATION

These steps have been prepared to help minimize or eliminate any issues when installing the Dentrix Learning Edition. For a successful installation, follow the steps below exactly. Please read through all the steps before attempting to install the Learning Edition.

1. Ensure System Meets the System Requirements

It is important for you to verify that your computer meets the current system requirements before you install the Dentrix Learning Edition. The System Requirements are listed below. The System Requirements describe the minimum standards for using the Learning Edition. Exceeding the minimum standards may result in better system performance.

Minimum system requirements:

- Operating system: Windows 7 Sp1, 8.1, 10 (Note: Dentrix Learning Edition supports any edition of Windows operating systems such as Home, Pro, Enterprise, etc.)

- Memory: 8 GB RAM

- CPU: 4 cores at 2.4 GHz

- Local drive install space: 40 GB total,

- 5 GB on C: drive

- Monitor: 1280 × 1024

How to check your available disk space:

- If you are using Windows 10: Right-click the Start icon on the Windows task bar and click Settings. In the Device Specifications section, look at the Installed RAM line to see the installed and usable disk space.

- If you are using an older version of Windows: From the Start menu, click My Computer. Right-click the C:\ drive icon and then click Properties. The Local Disk Properties dialog box appears, and the General tab displays the used and free disk space.

2. Follow the Installation Instructions

Follow the step-by-step instructions in this guide to install the Dentrix Learning Edition.

3. Finish the Installation Completely

Do not interrupt the installation process, even if it looks as though nothing is happening. You will be prompted when the installation is ready to continue. Terminating an installation prior to completion could prevent the software from working properly.

INSTALLING THE DENTRIX LEARNING EDITION

1. Go to the Evolve Resources site, and click on Dentrix Practice Management Software Learning Edition in the Student Resources. The download will begin when you click the link.

   When the download is finished, click the download file to start the installation.

The **Setup Status** screen appears.

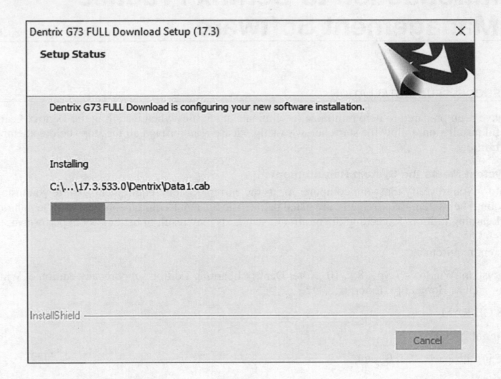

The **Preparing to Install** screen appears.

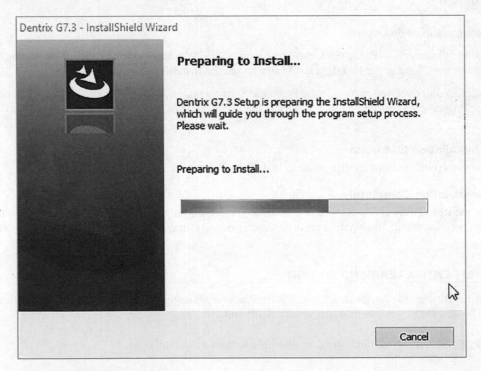

Introduction to Dentrix Practice Management Software

The **Select a Location** screen appears.

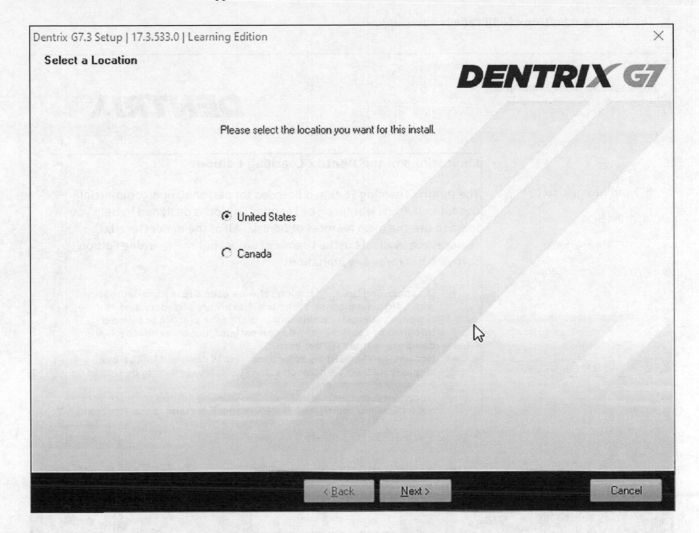

Dentrix G7.3 Setup | 17.3.533.0 | Learning Edition

Select a Location

DENTRIX G7

Please select the location you want for this install.

○ United States

○ Canada

< Back   Next >   Cancel

Introduction to Dentrix Practice Management Software

2. Choose your location (**United States or Canada**) and then click Next.

The **Important Software Notifications** screen appears.

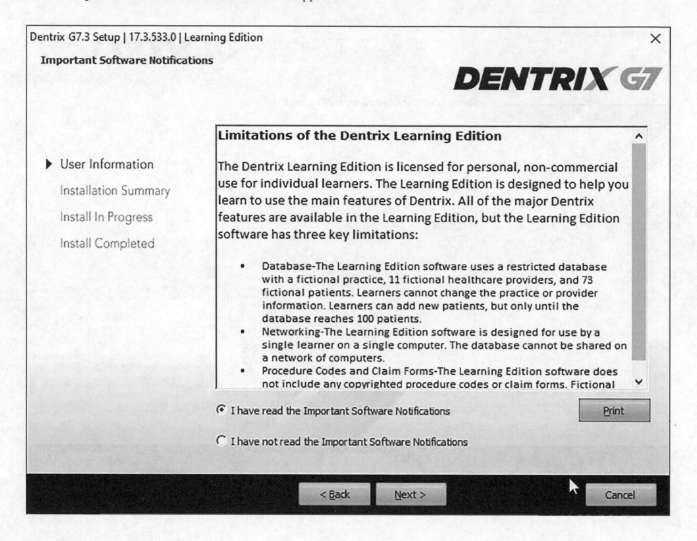

Introduction to Dentrix Practice Management Software

3. Read the notifications, select I have read the Important Software Notifications, and then click Next.

The **End User License Agreement** screen appears.

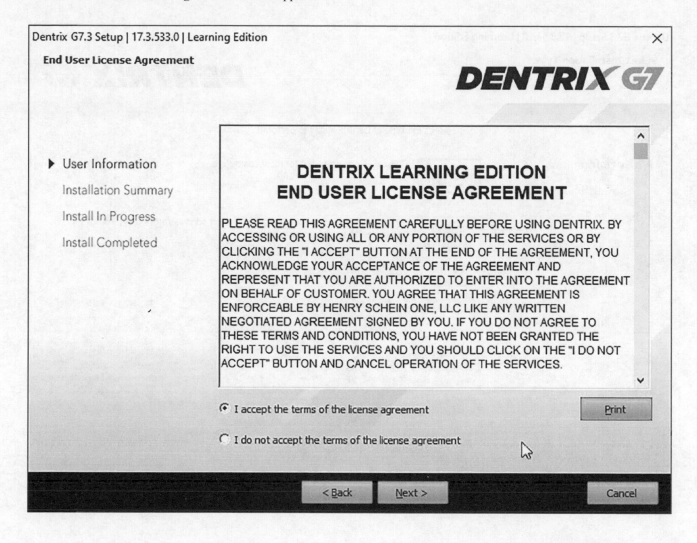

4. Read the agreement, select I accept the terms of the license agreement, and then click Next.

The **Select Installation Type** screen appears.

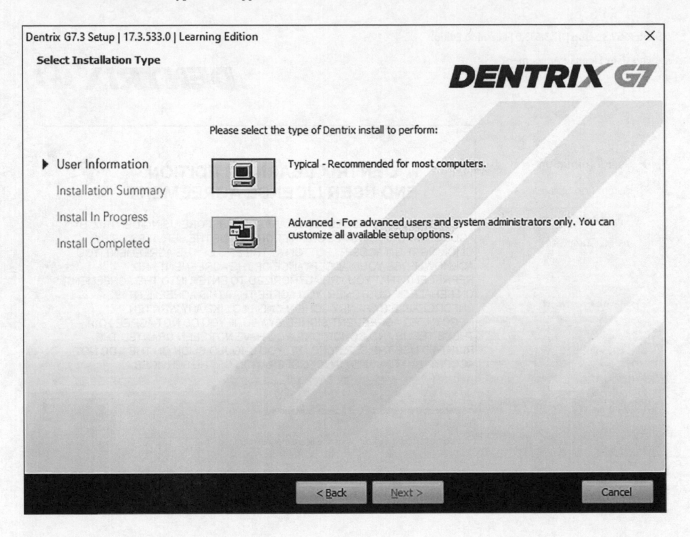

5. Click **Typical** as the type of installation you want to perform.

Dentrix will install all of the default Dentrix Learning Edition features. The Advanced option is for dental practices that are working with hardware technicians to install Dentrix on their network.

A system requirements check runs. If your system meets the requirements, the installation continues to the next step. If it does not meet the requirements, the **System Requirements Notice** dialog box displays what your system needs in order to meet the system requirements.

Dentrix G7.3 Setup | 17.3.533.0 | Learning Edition

Server Install

NOTICE: One or more of the Dentrix System Requirements are not met by this computer.

Component Description	This Computer	Required
✓ Processor	4 cores @ 2.80 GHz	4 cores @ 2.40 GHz
✓ Operating System	Microsoft Windows 10 Enterprise	Windows 7 SP1 / Server 2008 R2 SP1
✓ Operating System Architecture	64-bit	64-bit
✓ System Memory	7.88 GB	8 GB
✗ Network	0.65 Gbps	1 Gbps
✓ Drive Free Space (C:) : Data	309.63 GB	40 GB
✓ Drive Free Space (C:) : System	309.63 GB	5 GB
✓ Drive Free Space (C:) : Program	309.63 GB	4 GB

Do you wish to continue with the Dentrix installation using non-recommended components?

[No]   [Yes]

Note: A green check mark indicates that a component meets the requirements. A red "X" indicates that a component does not meet the requirements.

6. (Optional) If the **System Requirements Notice** dialog box appears, look at the report and do one of the following:

- To discontinue the installation and install the required components (recommended), click **No** to stop the installation.

- To continue the installation without meeting the recommended system requirements, type the phrase "I understand we may experience performance issues" exactly as it appears in the text box below the phrase. Click **Yes** to continue the installation.

The **Ready To Start Installation** screen appears.

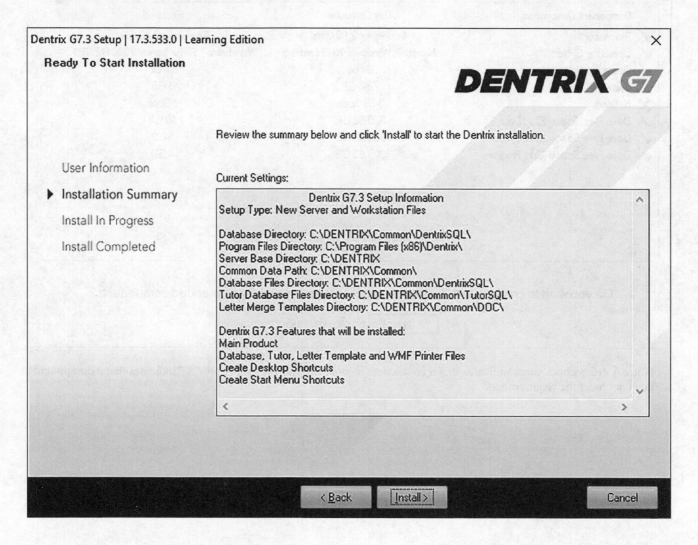

7. Click **Install**.

    The **Setup Status** screen appears.

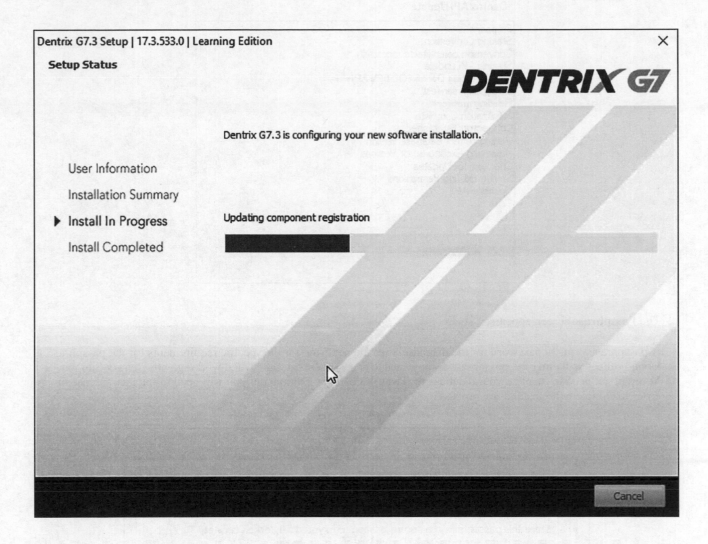

Introduction to Dentrix Practice Management Software

The **Dentrix API Update** dialog box appears.

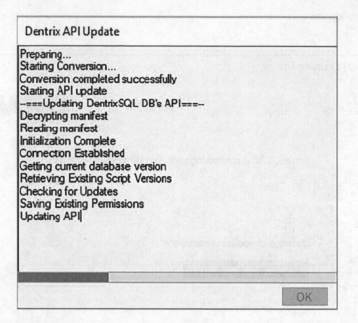

The **Passphrase** screen appears.

A passphrase is just a password for the database. (See the next step for the specific requirements for the passphrase.) Dental offices will enter the passphrase if they need to access their database when working with Dentrix Support. You will not need to manage your database for Dentrix Learning Edition, but you will need to set a passphrase in order to complete the installation process.

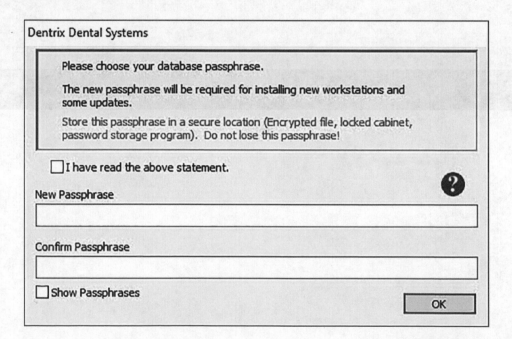

8. Do the following, and then click **OK**:

■ Read the message and select I have read the above statement.

■ Enter a passphrase that is at least 10 characters long and contains at least one of each of the following: a capital letter, a lower case letter, a number, and a special character (asterisk, question mark, or other character).

The **Letter Merge Add-in** screen appears.

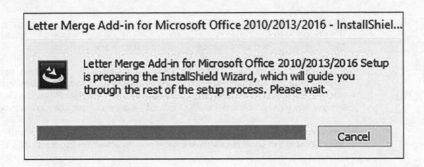

The **Setup Status** screen for required components appears.

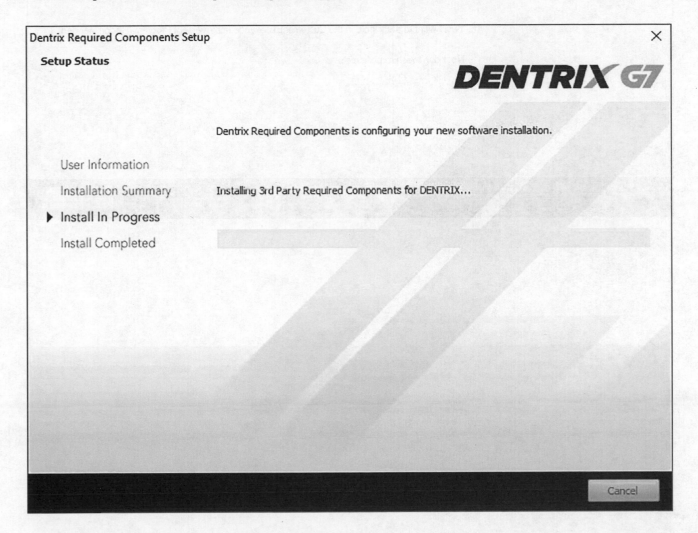

Introduction to Dentrix Practice Management Software

The **Customer Experience Improvement Progress** screen appears.

Dentrix Required Components Setup   ✕

Customer Experience Improvement Program

DENTRIX G7

User Information

Installation Summary

Install In Progress

▶ Install Completed

We invite you to participate in our Customer Experience Improvement Program to improve the quality, reliability, and performance of Dentrix software and services.

If you accept, we will collect information about your hardware configuration, how you use our software and services to identify trends and usage patterns and information related to any errors you may encounter when using the software. We will not collect Protected Health Information (PHI) or any other practice data. All of this will be done without interruption to your work.

You can leave this program at any time by clicking Help | About Dentrix from the Office Manager and checking the 'Disable Customer Experience Improvement Program' option.

⦿ Yes, I want to participate in the Customer Experience Improvement Program (Recommended)

○ No, I don't wish to participate

< Back   Next >   Cancel

9. Click **Yes** if you'd like to participate in the program or **No** if you do not want to participate.

The **Setup Complete** screen appears.

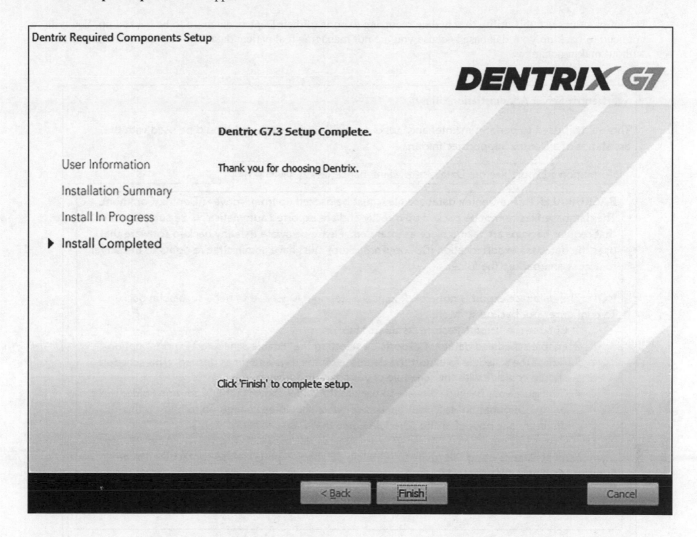

10. Click **Finish**.

The **Dentrix Server Administration Utility** appears.

Dental practices use this utility to schedule recurring exports of their Dentrix database to be backed up. You will not need to back up your database because you are not managing real patient data. You can just exit this utility without making changes.

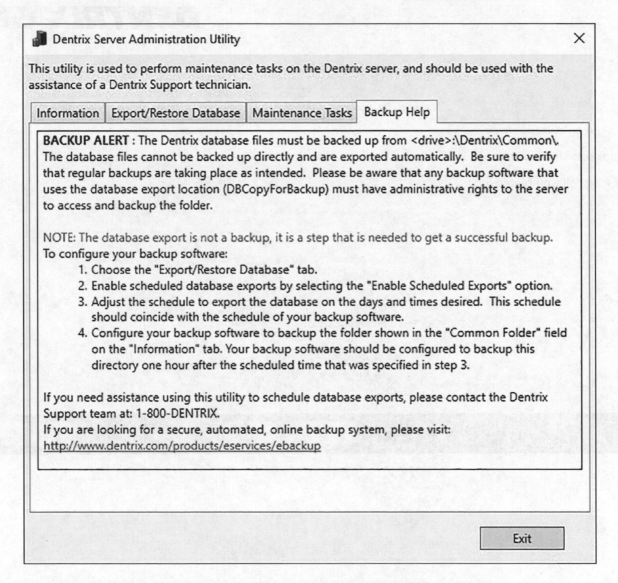

11. Click **Exit** without making changes in the utility. This will complete the installation process.

The InstallShield Wizard places shortcuts on your Windows Desktop, including those listed below. These shortcuts open Dentrix modules and give you access to the Dentrix G7 User's Guide.

- **Appointments:** Opens the Dentrix Appointment Book, the module you use to schedule patient appointments and manage your schedule.
- **Family File:** Opens the Dentrix Family File, the module you use to enter patient records and manage patient information.
- **Ledger:** Opens the Dentrix Ledger, the module you use to enter payments and manage accounts.

Introduction to Dentrix Practice Management Software

- **Office Manager:** Opens the Dentrix Office Manager, the module you use to run reports and set up practice defaults.

- **Patient Chart:** Opens the Dentrix Patient Chart, the module you use to chart treatment and enter clinical notes.

- **Dentrix Launcher:** Opens the Dentrix Launcher tool, which shows the Dentrix modules in the context of an office and helps you open the correct module for the task you want to perform.

- **Dentrix User's Guide:** Opens a PDF of the Dentrix G7 User's Guide.

Congratulations! You have installed your copy of the Dentrix Learning Edition.

RESOURCES FOR USING DENTRIX

If you need help, you can use any of the resources listed below.

On-Demand Training

Additional information, including on-demand software tutorials, can be found on the On-Demand Training web page. The tutorials explain fundamental concepts and guide you through hands-on practice exercises. You can even check your understanding with simple quizzes.

To access on-demand training, from any Dentrix module, click **Help > On-Demand Training**. If you have an Internet connection, the On-Demand Training web page opens.

Help Files

To access the Help files, open any module and click **Help > Contents**. The Dentrix Help window appears. In the Help, you can use the navigation tree on the Contents tab to find a feature in a specific module. Or you can type key words in the field on the Search tab to get a list of Help topics.

User's Guide

The Dentrix G7 User's Guide is saved on the Windows Desktop when you install the Learning Edition. With electronic documentation, you can quickly search for the information you need.

Dentrix Magazine

Dentrix Magazine is a quarterly publication that provides Dentrix news, tips and case studies to help Dentrix offices build more efficient and profitable dental practices. Visit http://dentrix.com/training/dentrix-magazine to visit the *Dentrix Magazine* page.

Facebook

Join the Dentrix fan community on Facebook. Get weekly tips about using Dentrix and chat with other Dentrix users. Log in to Facebook and "Like" Dentrix.

QUICK OVERVIEW OF DENTRIX

 Family File: The Family File module helps you manage each patient's name, address, employer, phone numbers, birth date, health history, insurance coverage, referrals, and other important information. Within the Family File, patients are organized by family. Each family must have a head-of-household (guarantor).

 Patient Chart: The Patient Chart module helps you manage the clinical information for patients. The Patient Chart allows you to post existing, completed, and recommended procedures. Additionally, the Patient Chart helps you keep detailed notes regarding patient care.

Several submodules of the Chart help users manage other clinical functions. The Presenter is a unique case presentation program that displays the treatment plan costs in terms of primary and secondary insurance portions and the estimated patient portion. The Perio Chart is one of the most comprehensive periodontal charting software tools available.

Ledger: The Ledger module helps you manage accounts. All financial transactions are recorded in the Ledger, including charges, payments, and adjustments. Additionally, from the Ledger, you can set up payment arrangements, file claims, and print statements.

 Office Manager: The Office Manager module provides you with day sheets, aging reports, and other financial reports. The Office Manager integrates with Microsoft Word, so you can create effective, professional-looking letters, appointment reminders, collection notices, and other documents. The Office Manager also helps you set up, customize, and maintain the Dentrix system.

 Appointment Book: The Appointment Book module helps you manage appointments. With the Appointment Book, you can search for available times, schedule appointments, record broken appointments, enter notes for daily tasks, and run a daily huddle report.

Orientation to the Dental Profession

LEARNING OBJECTIVES

1. Describe an effective dental healthcare team.
2. List the knowledge and skills that are expected of an administrative dental assistant.
3. List the personal traits and educational background of an administrative dental assistant.
4. Name the various members of the dental healthcare team and discuss the roles they play in the delivery of dental care.
5. Explain the rules and function of the Health Insurance Portability and Accountability Act of 1996 (HIPAA), including Administrative Simplification, as they apply to the dental healthcare system.
6. Describe the role of the Occupational Safety and Health Administration (OSHA) and the Center for Disease Protection (CDC) in dentistry.
7. Identify the five sections of the American Dental Association's *Principles of Ethics and Code of Professional Conduct* and demonstrate an understanding of its content by explaining, discussing, and applying the principles.
8. Explain the legal standards of dentistry, including licensure, registration, and certification.
9. Explain the rights of dental patients.
10. Describe the roles of the American Dental Assistants Association (ADAA) and the HOSA-Future Health Professionals.

INTRODUCTION

The dental profession in the 21st century is a complex healthcare delivery system. It uses the latest technology and demands caring, well-trained, multiskilled dental auxiliaries. The dental assistant is required to know all phases of the dental practice and the daily business operations. Those who excel and become vital members of the dental healthcare team will have mastered multiple skills, will be flexible, and will work well in a team environment.

EXERCISES

1. List the types of procedures and systems that are expected of an administrative assistant.

_____

_____

_____

_____

2. List examples of various software application used by an administrative assistant.

_____

_____

_____

_____

3. List examples of electronic messaging systems that may be used in a dental practice.

_____

_____

_____

_____

_____

_____

4. List the responsibilities of a dental receptionist.

_____

_____

_____

_____

_____

5. List the duties of a records manager.

_____

_____

_____

_____

6. Match the following job description with the appropriate administrative assistant:

a. _____ Typically will organize and oversee the daily operations of the office staff.

b. _____ Manages the fiscal operation of the dental practice, develops marketing campaigns, negotiates contracts, and oversees the compliance of insurance programs.

c. _____ Maintains all aspects of the patient's clinical chart according to preset standards.

d. _____ Responsible for entering data into the computer system.

e. _____ Organizes and maintains the daily schedule of patients.

A. Business Manager

B. Appointment Scheduler

C. Data Processor

D. Records Manager

E. Bookkeeper

F. Office Manager

G. Insurance Biller

7. List the personal traits of an effective administrative dental assistant.

_____

_____

_____

_____

_____

8. Refer to the traits you listed in Question 7, and select your strongest (or weakest) trait. Based on your selection, write a short paragraph (give an example) to support your selection.

_____

_____

_____

_____

_____

In the following scenarios, it will be the responsibility of the administrative dental assistant to refer the patient to a specialist. In the blank, identify the specialist you will refer the patient to for treatment.

9. Mrs. Tracy has been diagnosed with periodontal disease. Dr. Edwards instructs you to refer her to Dr. Usher for a

consultation. Dr. Usher is a(n) _____.

10. David Collins is a 4-year-old child with extensive dental caries. His mother has asked for the name of a dentist who

specializes in the treatment of children. You will refer David to a(n) _____.

11. Chris Salinas has been given the diagnosis of four impacted wisdom teeth. Dr. Edwards instructs you to refer Chris

to a(n) _____.

12. Judy Johnson was scheduled for an emergency visit. She has a tooth that is badly decayed. After Dr. Bradley exam-

ines Judy, he concludes that she will need a root canal. Judy will be referred to a(n) _____.

13. Mr. Kelly is an 85-year-old man who has been wearing dentures for a number of years. Because of extensive alveolar

bone loss on the mandibular arch, Dr. Edwards would like Mr. Kelly to see a(n) _____ because of the

complexity of the case.

14. Sally Davis is a 13-year-old girl with very crowded teeth. Dr. Edwards requested a referral to a(n) _____
for a consultation.

15. Mrs. Gonzales was scheduled for a biopsy of oral tissue. The biopsy was sent to a(n) _____ for evaluation.

16. Dr. Parker is the director and chief dentist in a government-sponsored inner city dental clinic. The specialty Dr. Parker

practices is _____.

17. Based on what you learned in this chapter, what do the following acronyms stand for?

DDS _____

DMD _____

OSHA _____

ADA _____

CDA _____

ADAA _____

DANB _____

HIPPA _____

EDI _____

CDT _____

IBR _____

HHS _____

PHI _____

ePHI _____

HITECH Act _____

CDC _____

PHE _____

18. What is the primary purpose of the Administrative Simplification provision of the HIPAA document?

_____

_____

_____

19. What is the Information Blocking Rule of the Cures Act? What does it prohibit?

_____

_____

20. List the four sets of HIPAA Standards and give a brief description of each standard.

    1.

    2.

    3.

    4.

21. What is a public health emergency?

_____

_____

_____

_____

_____

22. List the highlights of the HITECH Act.

_____

_____

_____

_____

_____

23. List and briefly describe the five principles of ethics identified by the ADA.

_____

_____

_____

_____

_____

24. Define the following terms:

Ethics:

_____

_____

_____

_____

Legal Standards:

_____

_____

_____

Dental Practice Act:

_____

_____

_____

INTRODUCTION TO EXERCISES

Computer Application Exercise

The objective of the computer application exercises is to provide a platform where you can apply basic computer skills to create, complete, and organize your student work. In this and the following chapters there will be assignments that will require you to go to the Evolve website and download assignment worksheets, fillable patent forms, and other useful information. In addition, you will also be directed to the Dentrix website to complete the Dentrix Learning Edition Lessons applicable to the chapter. These lessons have been developed by Dentrix to provide an interactive demonstration of various components of their practice management software.

Dentrix Learning Edition Lessons

The assignments for each chapter will serve as an introduction and tutorial for the Dentrix Application Exercises applicable to each chapter of the workbook. You will be directed to the Dentrix website where you will click on the assigned lesson, watch the video, and then complete the **Check Your Knowledge** assignment. When you complete the assignment, you will record the information on the Dentrix Learning Edition Assignment Sheet (you downloaded the form from the Evolve website in the previous assignment).

Dentrix Application Exercise

Dentrix Learning Edition software introduces you to a *real-world* dental practice management software and is designed to help develop basic skills. Dentrix is a leader in dental practice management software and dental office technology integration. The program that you will download is the Dentrix Learning Edition, a special version of Dentrix G7.3 designed specifically for educational purposes. It includes a preloaded database of patients and is interactive, allowing you to perform various tasks the way they are done in the dental office.

Student Learning Outcomes will clearly state what you will be able to do when all of the assignments have been successfully completed.

The Dentrix User's Guide Resources will direct you to sections of the User's Guide that will provide detailed information and instruction on the use of the software. In the previous exercise you downloaded the User's Guide and placed it in a folder on your computer for easy access. When you open the guide, you will find a table of contents. The table is organized by chapter followed by a list of the functions that will be explained in each chapter. The User's Guide is the full version for the G7.3 software, and all of the functions covered may not be accessed in the Learning Edition.

Dentrix Guided Practice is a series of tasks that will guide you through step by step, so you become familiar with the software. During the guided practice you may have **student assignments** that will ask you questions or instruct you to use specific information; these are designed to help you apply specific knowledge and skills.

Dentrix Independent Practice exercises will give you the opportunity to apply what you have learned to tasks that will be expected of an administrative assistant.

COMPUTER APPLICATION EXERCISE

Go to Evolve and download the assignments for Chapter 1

Student Assignment #1

You will create The Administrative Dental Assistant Workbook (ADA WB) electronic folder on your computer to organize and store your student work. In the following chapters you will add work to the chapter folders, retrieve downloaded fillable patient forms, access the Dentrix Users Guide, and more. Most importantly, you will be able to practice and apply skills that will be expected of you as an administrative assistant.

   Note: If you do not know how to create a folder, manage files, and place items in a folder, you will need to ask your instructor for help, google the question, or click the help button on your computer.

1. Create a folder on your computer and name it ADA WB.

2. Create a folder for each of the chapters in the workbook and name them Chapter 1, Chapter 2, and so on (1-18) and place them in the ADA WB folder.

3. Create folders for the following and place them in the ADA WB folder:

   a. Dentrix Learning Edition Lessons

   b. Dentrix User's Guide.

4. Go to the Evolve website and download the assignment for Chapter 1.

5. Complete the assignment.

6. Print a copy of the completed assignment and place a copy in your ADA WB Chapter 1 folder (this will be the folder you created in the exercise above).

Dentrix Learning Edition Lessons
Student Assignment #2

Go to the Evolve website and complete the Dentrix Learning Edition Lesson assignment for Chapter 1.
Lesson: Getting Started
   Opening Dentrix Learning Edition
   Dentrix Learning Edition Modules
   Selecting a Patient

DENTRIX APPLICATION EXERCISES

Before you can begin this exercise, it will be necessary to download the Dentrix G7 Learning Edition to your computer. Please review the instructions in the front of the workbook. You will also need to become familiar with the icons used to open various elements of the program such as Office Manager, Patient Chart, Family File, Appointments, Ledger, and the Dentrix *User's Guide*.

Dentrix Learning Outcomes

The student will:

■ Recognize icons and short cuts common to Dentrix

■ Access Practice Resource Setup and identify

   ■ Practice information

   ■ Providers

   ■ Staff

■ Access Operatory Setup and add a new operatory

■ Access Procedure Code Setup and edit fees and notes

- Access Fee Schedule Maintenance and edit a fee schedule
- Become familiar with the Dentrix Learning Edition Lessons and the Dentrix G7.3 User's Guide as resources for additional instruction, hands-on exercises, and assignments.

Dentrix User's Guide Resources

Chapter 1: Introduction and Initial Setup
    Dentrix Overview
    Opening Dentrix Modules
    Setting up Practice Resources

Dentrix Guided Practice

As a clinical and practice management software system, Dentrix manages a variety of information, including patient demographics, clinical details, scheduling, and production analysis. To simplify the process of entering and finding data, the Dentrix software is divided separate modules, each of which manages specific types of information and data.

Student Assignment #3 (information will be found in the front of the workbook and in the User's Guide)

List the five main modules and briefly describe the function of each.

1. _____

  _____

  _____

  _____

2. _____

  _____

  _____

  _____

3. _____

  _____

  _____

  _____

4. _____

  _____

  _____

  _____

5. _____

  _____

  _____

  _____

Practice Setup

With the Dentrix G7.3 Learning Edition, a default practice is set up for you in the Tutor database. In the Learning Edition you will be able to view and change some but not all of the information. When you attempt to edit information that is unchangeable, you will get an error notice. Click **OK** to close the message.

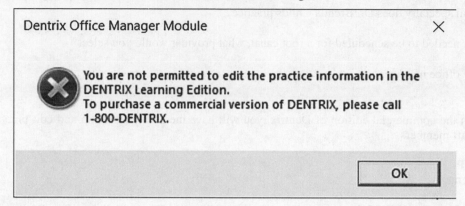

Provider and Staff Setup

To view the practice information, in the Office Manager, select **Maintenance-Practice Setup-Practice Resource Setup.** The Practice Resource Setup dialogue box appears. Answer the following questions with the information located in the **Practice Resource Setup** dialogue box:

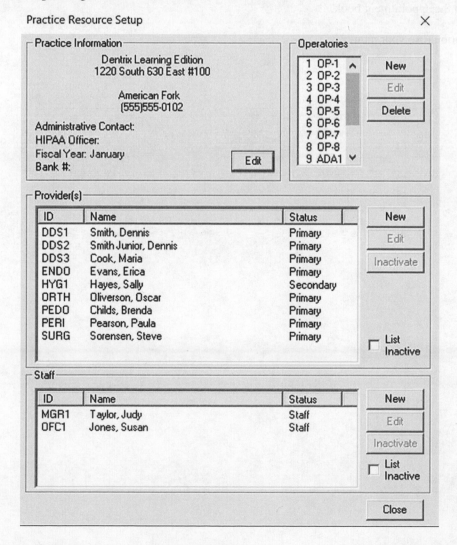

Student Assignment #4

1. What is the telephone # for the practice?

2. What dental specialty does Dr. Brenda Childs practice?

3. If a patient needed to be scheduled for a root canal, what provider would you select?

4. Who is the office manager?

Click **Close.**

Please note: With the commercial edition of Dentrix, you will have the ability to set up and edit practice information, providers, and staff members.

Operatory Setup

To add a new operatory:

1. In the Office Manager, select **Maintenance-Practice Setup-Practice Resource Setup**. The Practice Resource Setup dialogue box appears (see above).

2. In the Operatories group box, click **New.**

3. Enter an ID for the operatory in the **ID** field (enter the first four letters of your name). This information will appear as an operatory in the appointment book.

4. Enter a description (use your name).

5. Click **OK**

6. Click **Close.**

Procedure Codes Setup

You can set up new procedure codes to fit the needs of your office. The Learning Edition does not include the standard CDT codes. Because of copyright reasons, they have been replaced with non-ADA codes.

1. In the Office Manager, select **Maintenance-Practice Setup-Procedure Code Setup.** The Procedure Code Setup dialogue box appears.

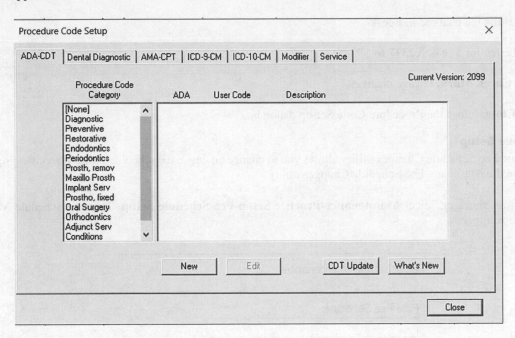

2. Click the **ADA-CDT Codes** tab Preventative and scroll through the Procedure Code Categories until you locate **X2397.**

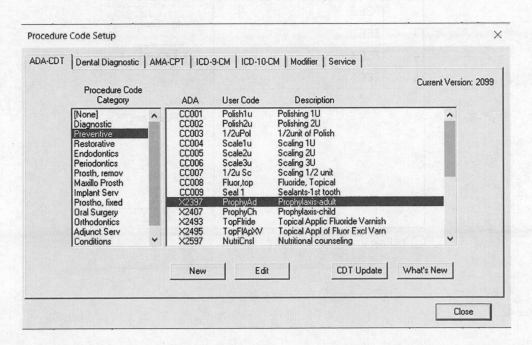

3. Click **Edit.**

Student Assignment #5
Answer the following questions:

1. What is the name of the dialogue box you just opened?

2. What is the *Description?*

3. What is the fee charged in **Fee 4**?

4. Edit the fee for **Fee 4, X2397 to** $93.00.

    Click the **Check Mark,** to save changes.

5. Click **Close.** (close the Procedure Code Set-up dialog box)

Fee Schedule Setup

The Automatic Fee Schedule Changes utility allows you to change an entire fee schedule rather than changing one fee at a time. To use the Automatic Fee Schedule Changes utility

1. In the Office Manager, select **Maintenance-Practice Setup-Fee Schedule Setup.** The Fee Schedule Maintenance dialogue box appears:

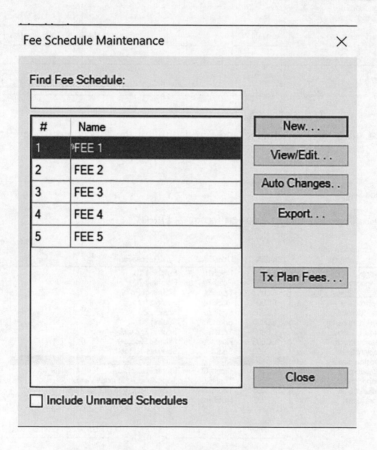

2. Select **Fee 4.**

3. Click **Auto Change.** The Automatic Fee Schedule Changes (Fee 4) dialog box appears

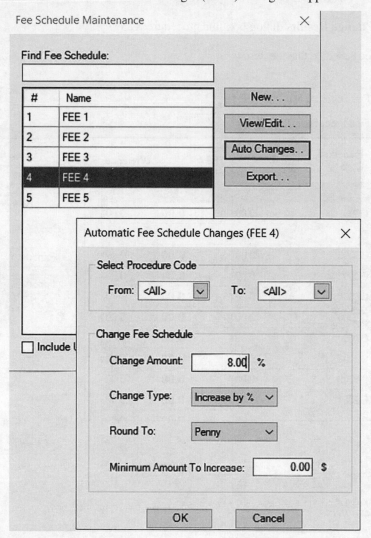

4. Increase the fees by 8%. **Change Amount** 8.00

5. **Round** to the dollar

6. Click **OK**

7. In the **Fee Schedule Change Results** dialog box find procedure X2397

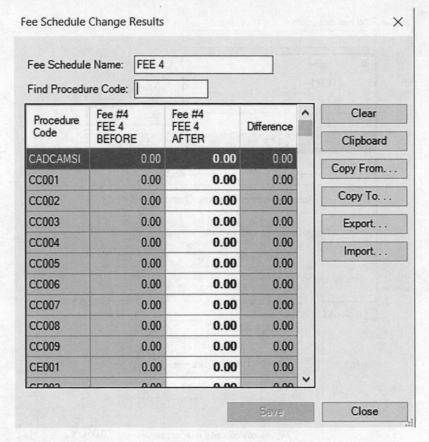

Student Assignment #6
Answer the following questions:

1. What was the **Before** fee for procedure X2397?

2. What is the new fee?

8. Click **Save**

9. Click **Close**

10. Click **Close** (Close the Fee Schedule Maintenance dialog box)

To review all the setup features in detail, refer to the Dentrix *User's Guide.*

2 Dental Basics

LEARNING OBJECTIVES

1. List the various areas of the dental office and explain the design and function of each area.
2. Label the basic structures of the face and oral cavity, including the basic anatomical structures and tissues of the teeth.
3. Label the primary and permanent dentition using the Universal, International, and Palmer numbering systems.
4. Chart dental conditions using an anatomical, geometric, and electronic charting system.
5. List and describe basic dental procedures.

INTRODUCTION

The administrative dental assistant has a unique opportunity to communicate in several "languages." You will be a translator between the dental community and the patient. As part of your job, you will represent the dentist when you communicate with dental professionals, dental insurance companies, patients, vendors, and fellow team members. Patients are often unwilling or unable to ask the dentist questions directly, so they will turn to the assistants for clarification. To be an effective communicator, you must first understand the language of dentistry.

EXERCISES

1. Identify the different areas of the dental practice.

   a. _____ The first area to be viewed by the patient.

   b. _____ Area used by administrative dental assistants to perform daily business tasks.

   c. _____ A private area used to discuss confidential information with a patient.

   d. _____ Area where duties pertaining to the fiscal operation of the dental practice take place.

   e. _____ Area where patients are treated by the dentist, dental hygienist, and dental assistant.

   f. _____ Consists of a contaminated area and a clean area.

   g. _____ Dental x-rays are taken in this area.

   h. _____ Dental radiographic film is processed in this area.

   A. Sterilization area

   B. Clinical area

   C. Reception area

   D. Business office

   E. Nonclinical areas

   F. Staff room

   G. Darkroom

   H. Treatment rooms

   I. Consultation area

   J. Radiology room

   K. Storage area

2. Label the following diagram:

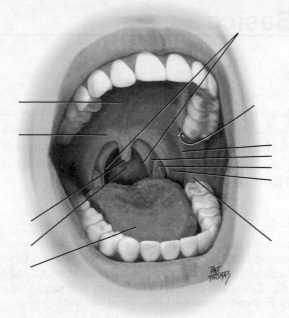

(From Fehrenbach MJ, Herring SW: *Illustrated anatomy of the head and neck,* ed 3, St. Louis, 2007, Saunders. © Pat Thomas, CMI.)

3. Label the following diagram:

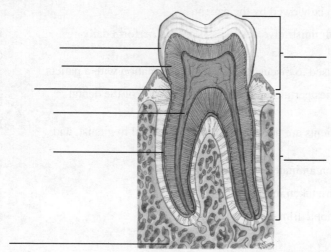

(From Bath-Balogh M, Fehrenbach MF: *Illustrated dental embryology, histology, and anatomy,* ed 3, St. Louis, 2011, Saunders.)

Using the patient chart below, complete the following tasks:

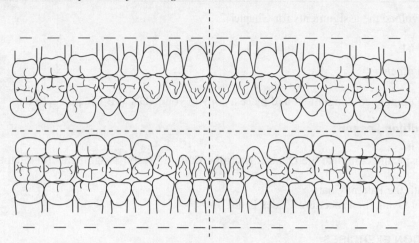

(From Bird DL, Robinson DS: *Modern dental assisting,* ed 10, St. Louis, 2012, Saunders.)

4. Correctly number the teeth on the chart (space provided on the chart above the maxillary arch and below the mandibular arch) using the Universal/National Numbering System.

5. Correctly chart the following conditions using the symbols described in Chapter 2 (use red and blue or black pencil):

   a. Maxillary right third molar, impacted

   b. Maxillary right second molar, MO restoration

   c. Maxillary right second premolar, MOD caries

   d. Maxillary right central, bonded veneer

   e. Maxillary left central, bonded veneer

   f. Maxillary left first molar, DO restoration

   g. Maxillary left third molar, missing

   h. Mandibular left third molar, missing

   i. Mandibular left first molar, full gold crown

   j. Mandibular left cuspid, periapical abscess

   k. Mandibular right lateral, mesial composite

   l. Mandibular right second premolar, occlusal caries

   m. Mandibular right first molar, completed endodontic treatment, post and core, PFM

   n. Mandibular right third molar, needs to be extracted

COMPUTER APPLICATION EXERCISES

Go to Evolve and download the assignments for Chapter 2.

Student Assignment #1

1. Complete the assignment

2. Print a copy of the completed assignment and place a copy in your ADA WB Chapter 2 folder.

Dentrix Learning Edition Lesson
Student Assignment #2

Go to the Evolve website and complete the Dentrix Learning Edition Lesson assignments for Chapter 2.
Lesson: Charting
   Getting Started with the Patient Chart
   Charting Treatment Using the Procedure Codes Panel

DENTRIX APPLICATION EXERCISES

Dentrix Student Learning Outcomes

The student will:

■ Post existing, recommended, and completed treatment or conditions in the Patient Chart.

■ Print a Patient Chart.

Dentrix User's Guide Resources

Chapter 5 Patient Chart

- ■ The Patient Chart Window
    - ■ Patient Chart Buttons
    - ■ Procedure Codes
    - ■ Status Buttons
- ■ Entering Treatments
    - ■ Adding Treatments from the Procedure Code Panel
- ■ Editing Treatment
- ■ Printing the Patient Chart

Dentrix Guided Practice
Posting Treatment to the Patient Chart
Keeping an electronic record of your patient's treatment is the primary way treatment is charted. In most dental offices the clinical dental assistant completes charting during the examination and records procedures after each dental visit. To help expand your skills, the following is a brief introduction to electronic dental charting.

The Administrative Assistant Workbook: Chapter 2

Student Assignment #3
Study the Patient Chart Window Section located in Chapter 5 of the Dentrix User's Guide and become familiar with how the Patient Chart is divided. You will also find more detailed information located in the "The Patient Chart overview" in the Dentrix **Help.**

To access Dentrix Help,

1. Open the Dentrix Patient Chart Module, click **Help**.

2. Select Contents…

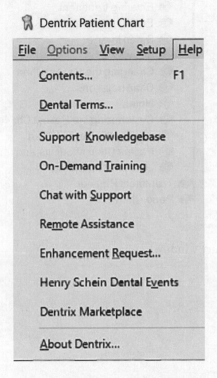

3. Click Patient Chart overview

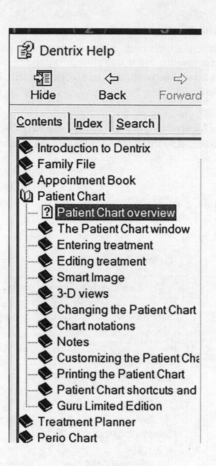

4. Scroll through and click **Patient Chart window**

5. Scroll through and click **toolbars**

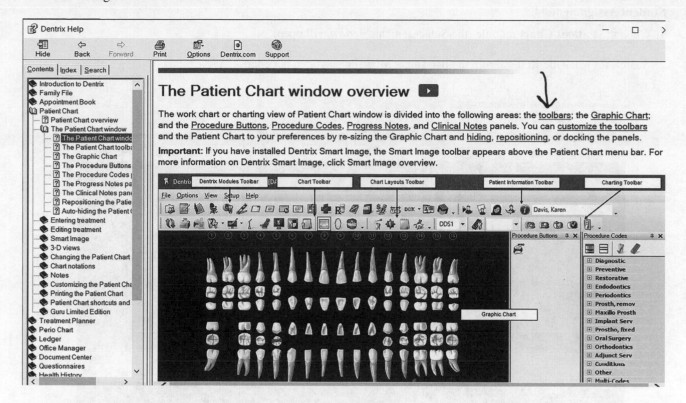

The Patient Chart Window has several toolbars. Briefly describe the function of each of the following toolbars.

1. Dentrix Modules Toolbar

2. Chart Modules Toolbar

3. Chart Layouts Toolbar

4. Patient Information Toolbar

5. Charting Toolbar

Posting Procedures in the Dentrix Patient Chart
Student Assignment #4

1. Click the **Patient Chart** module (the Select Patient window will open).

2. Search for Michelle Keller. From the list, select Michelle and open her chart.

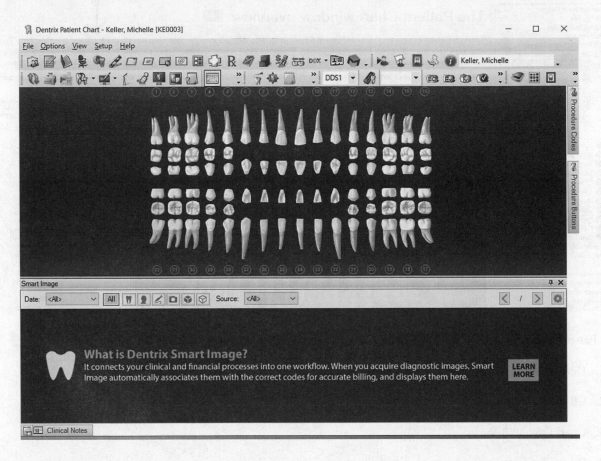

3. Close the **Smart Image** panel (if open).

4. You will be charting and existing DO amalgam restoration on tooth #2. **Select** tooth # 2 in the graphic chart.

5. Click the **Procedures Code** panel (the tab is located at the right-hand side of the chart).

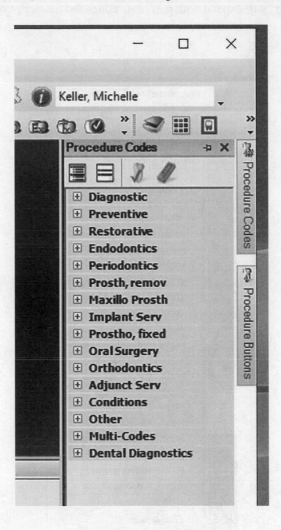

6. Select the procedure category from the Procedure Code panel (such as Diagnostic, Preventive, Restorative, and so on). Click **Restorative.** The list will expand with procedure codes and a description.

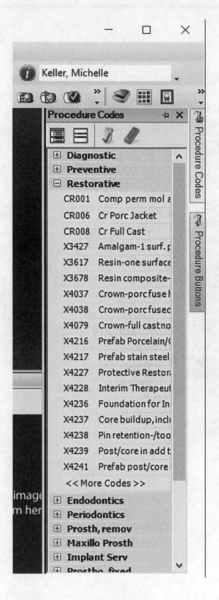

Tip: If the code is not listed, you may have to expand the list; scroll to the end of the list and click **more codes.**

7. Select the desired procedure X3437 Amalgam 2-surf. Prim/perm

8. Click the **Post** button (located at the top of the Procedure Codes Panel). Check and make sure the code is listed in the Procedure Code field.

9. Click the desired Status Button: Click **Existing (EX)**. The Select Surface dialog box appears.

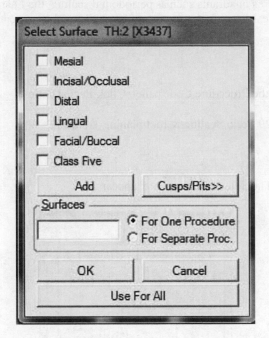

10. Check the desired surfaces, **Distal and Occlusal.**

11. Click **OK**

If everything was done correctly, you should see that tooth #2 on the Graphic Chart now illustrates a DO restoration in blue and the tooth is listed in the Progress Notes with a status of E. Click the **Progress Notes** button to view the progress notes.

Tip: To delete a procedure, highlight the desired procedure in the Progress Notes block and right click.

12. Close the **Progress Notes** and the **Clinical Notes** windows to return to the full Graphic Chart.

Entering Treatment for Multiple Teeth

Occasionally you may have the same procedure to enter for multiple teeth. This can be done by selecting all of the teeth on the Graphic Chart prior to entering the procedure code.

For this exercise you are going to enter that all four 3rd molars have been extracted (fully erupted) by a previous dentist.

Student Assignment #5

1. Select teeth numbers **1, 16, 17, and 32** in the Graphic Chart.

2. Click **Oral Surgery** in the Procedure Code panel.

3. Select procedure code X8057 Extraction Surgical/erupt. Tooth

4. Click **Post**. (Did the procedure code appear in the Procedure Code List field?)

5. Select Status. Click **Existing Other (EO)**.

Did the teeth disappear from the Graphic Chart? And is there a notation in the Progress Chart with a status of EO? If you answered YES, congratulations; if not, go back and try again.

Entering Treatment That Requires Quadrant(s)

If you select a procedure that requires quadrants such as periodontal scaling, the Learning Edition prompts you to select the applicable quadrants. For this exercise you are going to enter planned treatment for four quadrants of periodontal scaling.

Student Assignment #6

1. Select the procedure code from the Procedure Code panel. Click **Periodontics**.

2. Select the procedure code. X5629 Perio Scaling & root planing 1-3 quad.

3. Click **Post**.

4. Select Status button. Click **Tx**. The Select Quadrant box appears.

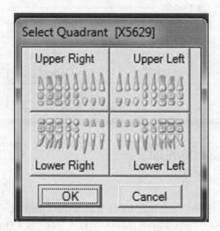

5. Select the quadrants. Click Upper Right, Lower Right, Upper Left, Lower Left.

6. Click **OK**.

Note: For this procedure you will not see anything post to the Graphic Chart, but you will see the procedures listed in the Progress Notes.

Student Assignment #7

1. On your own post the following treatment to Michelle's chart. Treatment plan a root canal (Endodontics X4617), post & core (Restorative, X4241) and porcelain fused to high noble crown (Restorative, X4037) for tooth number 30.

Tip: You can select all procedures in the Procedure Code panel before clicking the Post button.

2. Completed MOD composite for tooth number 29.

3. Existing distal resin to teeth numbers 8 & 9.

Printing a Patient Chart

If you want to give your patient a copy of their chart, you can print the Patient Chart.

Student Assignment #8

1. In the Patient Chart for your patient Michelle Keller, click the **Print Patient Chart** button. The Print Patient Chart dialog box appears.

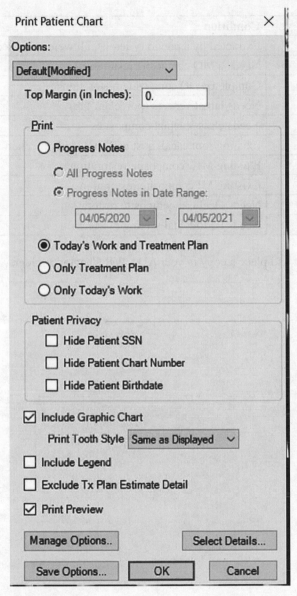

2. In the *Print* group box, mark the desired option. For this exercise, select:

   ■ Today's Work and Treatment Plan

   ■ Include Graphic Chart as Displayed

   ■ Print Preview

3. Click **OK**.

4. Preview the chart and check for completeness.

5. Click the **Print Button**, select your printer's name and click **OK** to print.

27

Dentrix Independent Practice

You have been asked to chart the following conditions for Pamela Schow. You will need to select the patient in the Patient Chart module, post the conditions, and print a copy of the patient chart to give to Pam.

Student Assignment #9

1. Enter the following conditions for Pamela Schow.

Tooth Number	Condition
1-16-17-32	Extracted by a previous dentist, all were impacted-soft tissue when extracted
3	Needs a MO composite restoration
4	Completed DO composite restoration
7-8-9-10	Needs labial veneers (porcelain-lab)
12-13-14	Needs class V labial composites
19	Existing root canal, post and core, and porcelain fused to high noble crown
22	Existing MID composite restoration
25	Existing MI composite restoration
30	Needs Occlusal composite restoration
UR, LR, UL, LL quadrants	Needs Periodontal scaling (4+ teeth)

2. Print a copy of the assignment and place a copy in your ADA WB Chapter 2 folder.

3 Communication Skills and Tools

LEARNING OBJECTIVES

1. Identify the five elements of the communication process.
2. Differentiate between verbal and nonverbal messages, including how the two are used to send and receive messages, and demonstrate how the dental healthcare team sends nonverbal cues.
3. Categorize the different types of interpersonal communication and describe how they are used in the dental profession.
4. Discuss the barriers to effective communication and express how members of the dental healthcare team can remove these barriers.
5. Describe how culture can be a barrier to effective communications and explain what a dental practice can do to minimize the barrier.
6. Describe some of the techniques that should be used when communicating with patients who have a disability (visual, hearing, speech, and cognitive).
7. List the responsibilities of the sender and receiver that contribute to effective communication.
8. Identify and describe professional telephone manners.

INTRODUCTION

Communication is a two-way process in which information is transferred and shared between a sender and a receiver. Communication can occur between individuals or groups. The four broad categories of communication are written, verbal, nonverbal, and visual.

Written communications include letters, e-mails, newsletters, patient documentation, and anything else that is typed or handwritten into words. **Verbal communication** is auditory (speaking and hearing) and includes speaking, music, sounds, and language. **Nonverbal communications** include body language (gestures and movement) and **visual communications** (pictures, charts, film, video, sign-language, dance).

During the communication process, information is transferred from one person or group to another through a system of symbols (written and spoken language), behaviors (tone of voice), and actions (nonverbal gestures). Transfer is effective only when information is shared and understood. Communication may seem like a very natural and simple task, but during transfer of information, several barriers can interfere with it. It is important for the dental healthcare team to understand and practice effective communication skills in any format.

EXERCISES

1. List the elements of the communication process that are linked together to complete the exchange of information. Demonstrate the process by writing a script or illustrating the process in a drawing and labeling the elements.

_____

_____

_____

_____

_____

29

_____

_____

_____

2. Verbal messages can be divided into two categories. Name each category and give two examples.

■ (Category) _____

   Example: _____

   _____

   Example: _____

   _____

■ (Category) _____

   Example: _____

   _____

   Example: _____

   _____

3. What positive nonverbal messages can be sent from a member of the dental healthcare team to the patient? List and give an example of how the nonverbal message can be conveyed.

   Nonverbal message: _____

   Example: _____

   Nonverbal message: _____

   Example: _____

4. What is visual communications?

   _____

   _____

5. Give examples of visual aids that may be found on a dental practice website (Hint: go to an actual dental practice website and list the items that are visual aids).

   _____

   _____

   _____

6. Interpersonal communication takes place when the sender and the receiver are exchanging information in real time. Match the type of transfer (typical to a dental practice) with the following statements:

   a. _____ Administrative assistant is instructed to call the pharmacy.

   b. _____ Patient calls to schedule an appointment for her children.

   c. _____ Hygienist gives oral hygiene instructions to a patient.

   d. _____ Office staff meeting is held.

   e. _____ Administrative assistant schedules patient's appointment.

   f. _____ Patient has a question concerning her statement.

   g. _____ Patient inquires about the types of dental insurance accepted.

   h. _____ Dentist consults with a specialist concerning the diagnosis and
   treatment plan of a patient.

   i. _____ Administrative assistant reviews financial arrangements with a
   patient.

   j. _____ Employee is given a performance review.

   A. Patient to Dental Healthcare Team

   B. Dental Healthcare Team to Patient

   C. Team Member to Team Member

   D. Professional to Professional

7. Identify the type of barrier to effective communication that may take place in the following situations:

   a. _____ "Mr. Franklin, you are scheduled for a filling." (administrative assistant)

   b. _____ "I am not sure, but I think you should feel all right when the doctor is finished today." (administrative assistant)

   c. _____ "I don't understand why the dentist wants to fix a baby tooth." (parent)

   d. _____ "I don't think you will want to have the treatment if your insurance company does not pay." (administrative assistant)

8. What is culture and how does it create a barrier to communications?

   _____

   _____

   _____

   _____

   _____

9. We need to show respect for people from other cultures and honor their values and beliefs. List three ways a dental practice can remove cultural barriers to communications in the dental practice.

   _____

   _____

   _____

   _____

10. When creating a positive telephone voice, it is important that you _____.

    a. develop an active script

    b. smile

    c. learn new phrases

    d. all of the above

11. A telephone should be answered within _____ rings.

    a. two

    b. three

    c. four

    d. five

12. When you are answering the telephone, your greeting should include all of the following except

    a. identify the practice by name.

    b. identify yourself by name.

    c. use good listening skills.

    d. time of day, for example, good morning, good afternoon.

13. Personal telephone calls are appropriate when

    a. you personally answer the telephone.

    b. you are not busy.

    c. you ask the dentist first.

    d. you have an emergency.

14. The HIPAA Privacy Rule states that you must take appropriate and reasonable steps to keep a patient's personal health information private. Please describe how you would do this in a dental office.

_____

_____

_____

WHAT WOULD YOU DO?

You are reviewing the charts for the next day and you notice that you have four patients who may need assistance completing their health history updates. How will you accommodate each of the following patients?

a. Mrs. Jones who is visually impaired.

_____

_____

_____

b. Mr. Smith who is hard of hearing.

_____

_____

_____

c. Ms. Frank with a developmental disability.

_____

_____

_____

d. Mr. Adams does not speak English.

_____

_____

_____

Computer Application Exercsis
Go to Evolve and download the assignments for Chapter 3.
Student Assignment #1

1. Complete the assignment.

2. Print a copy of the completed assignment and place a copy in your ADA WB Chapter 3 folder.

4 Written Correspondence and Electronic Communication

LEARNING OBJECTIVES

1. Discuss the four elements of letter writing style.
2. Describe letter style appearance as it applies to a finished business letter.
3. Identify the five basic letter styles and understand the different parts of a business letter.
4. Evaluate a completed business letter by judging letter style appearance, identifying letter style format, and assessing punctuation style.
5. Identify when Health Insurance Portability and Accountability Act (HIPAA) Privacy and Security Rules apply to written communications.
6. Describe the types of correspondence used in dentistry.
7. Create a professional e-mail message.
8. Describe the elements of a professional text message.
9. Discuss the various types of mail and determine how each type should be handled.

INTRODUCTION

Written correspondence is no longer limited to letters sent to patients and other professionals. Today, the progressive dental practice uses written communication to perform a wide variety of tasks, both paper based and digitally based. Computers are useful in a dental practice because they can be used to create printed and electronic communication. They can be used to develop patient brochures and monthly newsletters, create office manuals for employees, store databases and sample letters, and perform merge techniques to mass mail an assortment of letters and notices. In addition, computers are used to create and distribute web-based communications such as blogs, business Facebook pages, tweeter accounts, Instagram posts, and YouTube productions.

EXERCISES

1. Define the following letter writing elements of style:

   Tone: _____

   _____

   _____

   _____

   _____

   Outlook: _____

   _____

   _____

   _____

   _____

"You" technique: _____

_____

_____

Organization: _____

_____

_____

2. Compose one or two sentences that are examples of

Tone: _____

_____

_____

Outlook:_____

_____

_____

"You" technique: _____

_____

_____

3. Match each of the following statements with the correct title:

a. _____ Address of the party receiving the letter.   A. Subject line

b. _____ Alert the reader that there is more to the letter.   B. Signer's identification

c. _____ Describes what the next step or expected outcome will be.   C. Salutation

d. _____ Draws attention to the person you wish to read the letter.   D. Reference initials

e. _____ Draws attention to the subject of the correspondence.   E. Main body

f. _____ Final closing of the letter and is a courtesy.   F. Line spacing

g. _____ First paragraph and states the reason you are writing.   G. Letterhead

h. _____ Gives details of the points that you stated in the introduction.   H. Introduction

i. _____ Greeting.   I. Inside address

j. _____ Identifies the dental practice that is sending the letter.   J. Enclosure reminder

k. _____ Identifies the writer of the letter.   K. Date line

l. _____ Is used when the sender of the letter is representing the company.   L. Copy notation

m. _____ The date the letter was written.   M. Complimentary closing

n. _____ Includes three sections.   N. Company signature

o. _____ Used to identify the sender and the typist of the letter.   O. Closing

p. _____ Used to notify the reader that a copy of the document is being forwarded to another party.   P. Body of the letter

Q. Attention lines

4. All letter sections begin at the left margin, and proper spacing is applied between sections.

a. Full-Blocked

b. Blocked

c. Semi-Blocked

d. Square-Blocked

e. Simplified or AMS

5. Date line is on the same line as the first line of the inside address and is right justified. Reference initials and enclosure reminders are typed on the same line as the signer's identification and are right justified.

a. Full-Blocked

b. Blocked

c. Semi-Blocked

d. Square-Blocked

e. Simplified or AMS

6. Same as blocked with one change; paragraphs are indented five spaces.

a. Full-Blocked

b. Blocked

c. Semi-Blocked

d. Square-Blocked

e. Simplified or AMS

7. Margins are the same as full-blocked, with the exception of date line, complimentary close, company signature, and writer's identification.

   a. Full-Blocked

   b. Blocked

   c. Semi-Blocked

   d. Square-Blocked

   e. Simplified or AMS

8. Style is fast and efficient.

   a. Full-Blocked

   b. Blocked

   c. Semi-Blocked

   d. Square-Blocked

   e. Simplified or AMS

9. Define electronic communications and give examples of how it will be used in the dental practice.

   _____

   _____

   _____

10. Can e-mail replace standard mail delivery in a dental practice? Explain your answer.

    _____

    _____

    _____

11. What is the difference between text messages that are sent to friends and professional text messages?

    _____

    _____

    _____

12. In the following exercise convert the general message into a text for a friend and then a professional text message.

   Hint: you will need to add missing information such as names, dates, times, your name, and the name of the dental practice, reason for the message where applicable to complete the message.

General Message	Text Message for a Friend	Professional Text Message
a. Ask for a good time to get together (schedule an appointment)		
b. Ask them to call you		
c. Give directions to where you are going to meet		
d. Confirm the meeting		

Computer Application Assignments

For this assignment you will need to go the Evolve website and download the documents for Chapter 4

Student Assignment #1

1. Complete the following tasks using the information below:

   Joel is being referred to Donald Payne, DDS, 23454 Tenth Street, Suite 234, Canyon View, California 91786, Attention Joan. The referral is for the extraction of teeth numbers 1, 16, 17, and 32. Joel is 18 years old and will be leaving for college in 3 weeks.

   Write a referral letter. (Use the letter head you downloaded from the Evolve website)

   a. Select a letter style of your choice.

   b. Use your initials in the reference initials.

   c. At the bottom of the page add your name, the date, and the letter style you used (for identification purposes).

2. Address the envelop (use the enveloped you have downloaded).

3. What letter style did you use? _____

4. Print a copy of the completed letter and envelop and place a copy in you ADA WB Chapter 4 folder.

WHAT WOULD YOU DO?

Student Assignment #2
You have been asked to create a guideline for the dental office on sending e-mail messages. In your guideline you need to cover the type of messages that should be sent via e-mail, examples of good subject lines, and how to get the response you want. Also, identify what information can be sent over an unsecured e-mail server and what types of messages need to be secure.
   Hint: Do an Internet search on "how to write an effective e-mail."

1. Type your guidelines.

2. Print a copy of the completed assignment and place a copy in your ADA WB Chapter 4 folder.

5 | Patient Relations

LEARNING OBJECTIVES

1. Compare and contrast the humanistic theory according to Maslow and Rogers. Relate the theory to patient relations.
2. Evaluate the purpose of Emotional Intelligence in the workplace.
3. List the different stages that present a positive image for the dental practice.
4. Describe the elements of a positive image and give examples.
5. Demonstrate different problem-solving techniques.
6. Examine different methods of providing outstanding customer service. Discuss team strategies and personal strategies for providing exceptional patient care.

INTRODUCTION

Patient relations involve empathy, understanding, concern, and warmth for each patient. These emotions can be demonstrated in the way we communicate with patients, in the type of service we provide, in how members of the dental healthcare team relate to each other, and in how problems are solved. Every aspect of the dental practice should be conducted with the understanding that the patient is "number one."

EXERCISES

1. Match the following statements with the corresponding stage:

   a. _____ Social media   A. Investigation Stage

   b. _____ Amount of information given   B. Initial Contact Stage

   c. _____ Answers to questions match individual needs   C. Confirmation of Initial Impression Stage

   d. _____ Appearance of the reception area   D. Final Decision Stage

   e. _____ Attitude and professionalism meet expectations

   f. _____ Communication skills of the staff and dentist

   g. _____ Financial arrangements meet needs

   h. _____ How the telephone is answered

   i. _____ Online Presence

   j. _____ Office is easy to find

   k. _____ Talking with friends

   l. _____ Time spent waiting

2. What is online presence and how were the identities created?

_____

_____

_____

_____

3. What can be done to ensure that patients' expectations are being met? List the seven points (summarize).

_____

_____

_____

_____

_____

_____

_____

_____

In the following scenario, the administrative dental assistant is faced with a typical daily problem. Michele Austin is a 32-year-old patient who has been scheduled three different times for completion of a root canal. Each time when you call and confirm the appointment, she finds some reason to postpone it. She has told you that her schedule at work is very busy and she cannot leave, that her daughter has a dance recital, and that she has to make final arrangements for the family dinner party. You have just called her for the fourth time, and this time she informs you that she will be leaving on vacation next week and wants to wait until she gets back.

4. What steps would you take to identify the problem? (With information given in the scenario, use your imagination and list the problem or problems.)

_____

_____

_____

_____

_____

_____

_____

_____

40

Chapter **5** **Patient Relations**

5. Based on your selected problem, what steps will you take to solve this problem? Is there more than one way to solve the problem?

_____

_____

_____

_____

6. Can the problem be prevented in the future? If so, how?

_____

_____

_____

_____

7. Identify strategies that can be used by the dental healthcare team to provide outstanding customer (patient) service.

_____

_____

_____

_____

_____

_____

8. Based on your personal experiences, which is the most important of these strategies (from Question 6), and why?

_____

_____

_____

_____

_____

_____

What Would You Do?

Student Assignment #1

You have been asked to work with a small team of colleagues (clinical assistant, dental hygienist, and associate dentist) to explore the development of a practice website. The practice is opening a new location, and the primary purpose of the site is to introduce the dental practice to the community. You have been asked to give your opinion on the following:

Type your response to following (include your name and date at the top of the page).

1. What do you think should be included on the website?

2. What are the legal and ethical advertising guidelines the dental practice needs to follow?

3. Provide examples (and links) of websites that meet your criteria and explain why.

Hint: Do an Internet search for "dental websites" and search the American Dental Association (ADA) website for advertising information.

4. Print a copy of the completed assignment and place a copy in your ADA WB Chapter 5 folder.

6 | Dental Healthcare Team Communications

LEARNING OBJECTIVES

1. Discuss the purpose of a dental practice procedural manual and identify the different elements of the manual.
2. Categorize the various channels of organizational communication and identify the types of communication that are used in each channel.
3. Identify and discuss barriers to organizational communications.
4. Describe different types of organizational conflict and select the appropriate style for resolution.
5. Explain the purpose of staff meetings.

INTRODUCTION

A team can be described as a group of two or more persons who work toward a common goal. Similar to those on a sports team, all members must understand and practice established rules and have a common goal. An effective healthcare team requires a shared philosophy, excellent communication skills, the desire to grow and change, and the ability to be flexible while providing quality care for all patients.

EXERCISES

1. List the main elements of a procedural manual.

   _____

   _____

   _____

   _____

   _____

2. Identify the four channels of organizational communication, and give two examples for each channel.

   _____

   _____

   _____

   _____

   _____

Identify the type of barrier to organizational communication that may result in the following scenarios:

3. Kim tells the office manager about a new idea she has that will improve the insurance billing process. The office manager decides not to tell the dentist about the idea. Classify the barrier. _____

4. Julie has a very full schedule as the receptionist. Kim, the insurance clerk, calls in sick and tells Julie that the daily insurance claims must be processed by the end of the day and asks if she will take on the responsibility of completing the task. Classify the barrier. _____

5. Kim is told that she will not get paid for her sick day because she did not report the absence correctly. Kim questions the ruling because it is the first time she has been informed that there is a reporting policy. Classify the barrier.

_____

6. Julie is excited about a new seminar that is being offered. She tries to explain the seminar to the dentist on his way out of the office to meet with the accountant. She is disappointed when he does not share in her excitement.

Classify the barrier. _____

7. Organizational conflict can be described as _____ (conflict within the organization) and _____ (conflict between two or more organizations).

8. Define the four types of intraorganizational conflict.

■ Intrapersonal Conflict:

_____

_____

_____

■ Interpersonal Conflict:

_____

_____

_____

_____

■ Intragroup Conflict:

_____

_____

_____

■ Intergroup Conflict:

_____

_____

_____

9. Identify and define the five conflict-handling styles, according to Rahim and Bonoma.

_____

_____

_____

_____

_____

What style of conflict resolution would be appropriate for the following problems (support your answer)?

10. Problem: A new computer system is needed.

_____

_____

_____

_____

11. Problem: You don't like the color of the new uniform, and everyone else thinks it is great. (You will have to wear this color only once a week.)

_____

_____

_____

_____

12. Problem: Dr. Edwards takes 2 weeks off during the summer and closes her office. Her staff cannot agree on a vacation schedule for all of them; therefore, Dr. Edwards sets the date and does not offer any options.

_____

_____

_____

_____

13. Problem: Julie and Kim both want to leave early to get ready for the long weekend. One person will have to stay until 6 PM to check out the last patient. Julie agrees to stay only if Kim will open for her on Tuesday morning.

_____

_____

_____

_____

14. State the purpose of a staff meeting at the beginning of each day.

_____

_____

_____

_____

COMPUTER APPLICATION EXERCISES

Student Assignment #1

1. Develop and type an agenda for your next staff meeting following the guidelines in the textbook. *Hint: google how to write an agenda for ideas on how to format an agenda.*
   Information for your agenda: (you may need to add additional information to complete your agenda depending on the type of meeting and other topics you think are relevant)

   - Location - your school

   - Facilitator - yourself

   - Date - today's date

   - Time - 8:00 AM

   - New business - Write the dress code for the procedural manual.

Hint: Use the information you completed in the "What Would You Do" exercise in the textbook.

2. Print a copy of completed agenda and place an electronic copy in your ADA WB Chapter 6 folder.

DENTAL PRACTICE PROCEDURAL MANUAL PROJECT (OPTIONAL)

The dental practice procedural manual is a detailed manual that is used as a form of written communication. The objective of the manual is to provide a reference for all team members. This resource provides each team member with specific details on practice goals, personnel procedures, business office procedures, and clinical procedures. The manual should be developed as a team project, with each team member contributing in his or her specific area of expertise. As procedures change, it is the team members' responsibility to update the manual. To be effective, the manual must be updated at regular intervals and all team members must be given updated manuals.

The key to developing a good procedural manual is to include as much information as possible without making the manual cumbersome. The idea is for the manual to be a resource for all team members. It will not be used on a daily basis by experienced team members, but it will be used to help train new team members and will serve as a guide for substitute team members or, when necessary, for a team member who fills in for another. The purposes of the manual are to provide written documentation of and to eliminate inconsistency in policies. Such inconsistencies are a common cause of conflict among members of the dental healthcare team.

Project Overview

During this project, which spans the full textbook, your team will do research, have discussions, and come to consensus about the information you will include in your procedural manual. The majority of the information your team will need will be in the textbook and created during Career Ready Practices exercises at the end of each chapter. In addition, you will need to do some research to find additional information.

How to approach the project:

1. Work as a team (although the project is designed as a team activity, it can be completed by individuals).

2. Name your dental practice.

3. Identify the roles and responsibilities of each team member. Develop a timeline to complete the project. How will the work be divided? How will the team discuss key issues? How will you resolve conflict?

4. Build upon previous activities presented in the text, for example, Career Ready Practices exercises, and What Would You Do scenarios.

5. Review procedural manuals from dental practices for ideas. You can obtain some online or ask a local dental practice for a copy of their manual. Remember, these are only samples; some may be very good while others may be outdated or missing information.

6. Your manual will have key components but will not have all the information that should be included in a comprehensive procedural manual. Feel free to expand upon the project and add components and information that is important to your team.

7. Remember, you want the manual to be easy to read; for example, information on procedures and job description can be as simple as an overview and a bulleted list.

8. Components of your manual can be completed at the end of the applicable chapter.

9. The finished procedural manual will be word processed and neatly organized. The final project may be used for the team grade.

10. Each team member will keep a journal about his or her role during the project to identify his or her responsibilities, major contributions, and time spent. This journal may be used for an individual grade.

11. Create a folder, *Dental Practice Procedural Manual Project,* and place it in your electronic ADA WB. You may want to subdivide the folder into other subjects to manage and organize your project.

Key Components for the Dental Practice Procedural Manual Project

The following components are a portion of what will be included in a comprehensive procedural manual. Some of the components are covered in several chapters throughout the textbook and may not be completed at one time, for example, job descriptions; although an overview of the job is given in Chapter 1, the detail will be covered in many other chapters.

Procedural Manual Section	Key Component	Primary Source Chapter
Practice Philosophy	Mission Statement	Chapter 1
General Instructions	Mission Statement for the Manual (team mission)	Chapter 6
How to Use the Manual	Chapter 6	
Responsibility for Updating and Reviewing	Chapter 6	
Personnel Procedures	Hiring	Chapter 18
Work Schedules	Chapter 10	
Job Descriptions	Several chapters	
Code of Conduct	Chapters 1-6	
Reviews and Evaluations	Chapter 18	
Termination Procedures	Chapter 18	
Health Insurance Portability and Accountability Act (HIPAA) Procedures	Identify Who Manages HIPAA Compliance	Chapter 1
Establish a Plan for Compliance	Chapter 1	
Identify the Components of HIPAA	Chapter 1, covered in several chapters	
Describe the Roles and Responsibilities of Various Members of the Dental Health Care Team	Chapter 1, covered in several chapters	
Mandated State and Federal Requirements	Health and Safety	Chapter 12
Electronic Health Records	Chapter 8	
Business Office Procedures	Specific Duties and Job Descriptions (detailed information for each procedure and duty performed in the business office)	Covered in several chapters
Records Management Protocol (detailed information for each type of record)	Chapter 8	
Clinical Area Procedures	Description of the Inventory Procedure	Chapter 12
Description of the Hazardous Material Program	Chapter 12	

Computerized Dental Practice

LEARNING OBJECTIVES

1. Compare the basic and advanced functions of dental practice management software and discuss their application.
2. Explain how to select a dental practice management system and list the functions to consider during the selection process.
3. Discuss the role of the administrative dental assistant in the operation of a computerized dental practice.
4. Identify the daily computer tasks performed by the administrative dental assistant, including the importance of a computer system backup routine.

INTRODUCTION

The computerized dental practice management system is an integrated system of software or application suites that are seamlessly linked to perform related functions. These powerful software suites connect the dental business office to the clinical treatment area and eliminate the need to store patient information on paper. The systems can also be cloud based, allowing multiple sites to share the same information. At its basic level, the software should store patient records, the practice schedule, and all business. Advanced capabilities can be added, such as digital imaging, integrated workstations, insurance processing, and patient communications. The ability to customize desired functions is key to enhancing patient care and increasing the dental practice's profitability.

EXERCISES

1. Briefly describe how information is gathered to build a patent's EHR.

_____

_____

_____

_____

_____

_____

_____

_____

_____

2. What are the basic business functions of a computerized practice management system?

_____

_____

_____

_____

3. What are the advantages of the additional tools and resources that are provided in more advanced software suites?

_____

_____

_____

_____

4. List the functions you should consider when selecting dental management practice software.

_____

_____

_____

_____

_____

_____

_____

5. Under the 21st Century Care Act patients have the right to view their electronic health information. What technology can be used to accommodate the patient's request? How else can the same technology be used to in the dental practice?

_____

_____

_____

6. In your opinion, what are two reasons a computerized practice management system is important to a dental practice?

_____

_____

_____

Describe the functions of the computerized practice management system that are of use to each of the following members of the dental healthcare team:

7. Accountant: _____

8. Dental hygienist: _____

9. Administrative dental assistant: _____

10. Insurance biller: _____

11. Describe the role of the administrative dental assistant in the operation of a computerized dental practice.

_____

_____

_____

_____

_____

12. What are the advantages of using a computerized system?

_____

_____

_____

_____

13. List the daily procedures performed with the use of computerized dental software.

_____

_____

_____

_____

_____

_____

14. Describe the importance of backing up a computerized dental practice system.

_____

_____

_____

_____

_____

15. Match the following computerized dental practice software terms to their definitions:

a. _____ Will appear when additional input is needed   A. Menu Bar

b. _____ Identifies software being used   B. Power Bar

c. _____ Gives you information about the screen you are currently working in C. Dialog windows or boxes

d. _____ are used to arrange the parts of a screen into a logical order   D. Search Button

e. _____ Icons configured as buttons that identify commonly used features   E. Tabbed Screen

f. _____ Lists the categories of options available to the user   F. Title Bar

g. _____ Provides quick access to selected features   G. Toolbar

h. _____ A list of options available under each category on the menu bar   H. Drop-Down Menu

COMPUTER APPLICATION EXERCISES

Student Assignment #1
Go to the Evolve website and download the assignment for Chapter 7.

1. Complete the assignment.

2. Print a copy of the completed assignment and place an electronic copy in your ADA WB Chapter 7 folder.

Dentrix Learning Edition Lesson
Student Assignment #2
Go to the Evolve website and complete the Dentrix Learning Edition Lesson assignments for Chapter 7.
Lesson: Patient Records
   Getting Started With the Family File

DENTRIX APPLICATION EXERCISE

Dentrix Student Learning Outcomes
The student will

- Identify key elements of the **Family File**

- Access patients by name and chart number

- Edit patient information such as address and telephone number

User's Guide Resources

Chapter 3: Family File

- The Family File Window
- Selecting Patients

Dentrix Guided Practice

One of the key features of any practice management system is how patient files are managed. In the Dentrix Learning Edition program, this is done in the Family File. The Family File manages and stores both patient and family information, such as address, phone number, insurance coverage, and medical alerts. Before you can perform many of the functions, you are required to select a patient.

Selecting a Patient

1. In the Family File, click the **Select Patient/New Family** button. The Select Patient dialogue box appears.

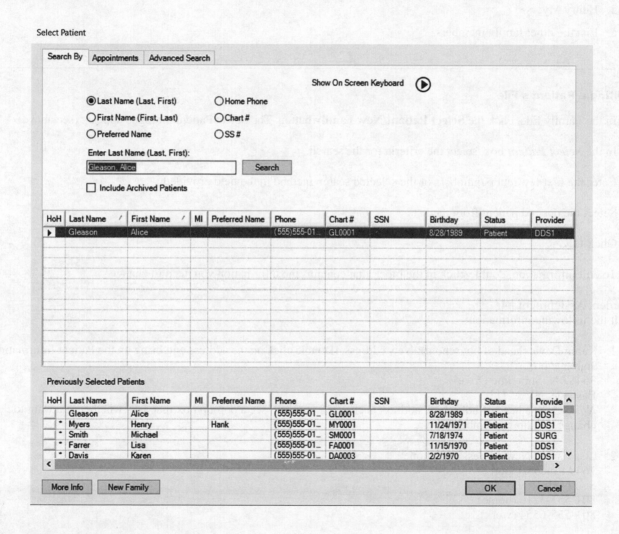

2. In the *Select Patient* box, select the criteria for the search.

3. Enter the first few letters/numbers of the selected search method in the field provided.

4. Select the desired patient from the list.

5. Click **OK.**

Student Assignment #3

Search for the following patients:

1. Alice Gleason

   a. What is Alice's chart number?

   _____

2. Chart #KE0004

   a. Who is the patient?

   _____

3. Henry Myers

   a. List the other family members.

   _____

Editing a Patient's File

1. In the Family File, click the **Select Patient/New Family** button. The Select Patient dialogue appears (see above).

2. In the *Select Patient* box, select the criteria for the search.

3. Enter the first few letters/numbers of the selected search method in the field provided.

4. Select the desired patient from the list.

5. Click **OK.**

6. To edit information, double click in the block that contains the information you need to change.

Student Assignment #4

Edit the following information:

1. Karen Davis (head of household): New address. (Double click on the address and bring up the Patient Information dialogue box.)
   36487 N. Shoreline Drive
   Eastside, NV 11111
   Note: Once a head of household address is changed, you will see a pop-up box that asks whether you want to change all family members.

2. Lisa Farrer: New address and phone
   7649 Lincoln Court
   Southside, NV 33333
   801-555-3210 (home)
   801-555-6554 (work)

3. Michael Smith: New address
   231897 Northwestern Avenue
   Centerville, NV 55555

DENTAL PRACTICE PROCEDURAL MANUAL PROJECT (OPTIONAL)

Continue working on your Dental Practice Procedural Manual (see Workbook Chapter 6 for details).
Suggested activities:

- Team meeting
- Review timeline
- Review Group research and writing assignments
- Complete research and writing assignments for this chapter
- Review and revise completed sections of the manual
- Individual journal entries

8 Patient Clinical Records

LEARNING OBJECTIVES

1. List the functions of patient clinical records and the key elements of record keeping. Describe the significance of each element.
2. Describe the two different methods of dental clinical record keeping.
3. List the types of information found in a dental clinical record and explain why the information is considered necessary.
4. Discuss methods used in the collection of information needed to complete clinical records.
5. Discuss the purpose of risk management and identify situations that lead to patient dissatisfaction.

INTRODUCTION

The function of the clinical record (electronic or paper) is to provide the dental healthcare team with information. The objective of the dental healthcare team is to deliver dental treatment that takes into consideration the needs of the patient. The whole picture cannot be correctly visualized if all of the pieces are not present. The information collected during preparation of the clinical record, when complete, provides all of the necessary pieces.

EXERCISES

1. What is the function of the following components of a clinical record?

   a. Registration form

   _____

   _____

   b. Medical History

   _____

   _____

   c. Dental History

   _____

   _____

   d. Treatment Plan

   _____

   _____

2. List the key elements of record keeping and describe the significance of each element.

   _____

   _____

   _____

3. What is an EHR?

_____

_____

4. Identify the components of a clinical record.

a. _____ An instrument used to communicate information about a patient.

b. _____ Provides demographic and financial information.

c. _____ Documents probing, bleeding, mobility, and furcation conditions.

d. _____ Outlines the work that is going to be done, describes reasonable results, and alerts the patient to complications that may result.

e. _____ Necessary to document the medical needs as well as the dental needs of the patient.

f. _____ Created each time an entry is recorded in the patient chart.

g. _____ is where existing, recommended, completed treatment or conditions are entered and charted.

h. _____ Plan derived from information collected in the clinical record.

i. _____ Must be signed by the patient or representative.

j. _____ places in writing the total estimated cost of the dental treatment, when payments are expected, and the amount of each payment.

A. Clinical Record

B. Treatment Plan information

C. Registration information

D. Recall Examination Form

E. Progress Notes

F. Perio chart

G. Medical History

H. Financial Arrangements

I. Patient chart

J. Consent Forms

K. Acknowledgment of Receipt of Privacy Practices Notice

5. Identify the components of the patient clinical record that are necessary forms.

_____

_____

_____

_____

_____

6. What is the purpose of patient authorizations? Give two examples

_____

_____

_____

7. What does the acronym TCPA stand for and how does the act apply to dentistry?

_____

_____

_____

8. Risk management is a process that

   a. organizes clinical records.

   b. is mandated by state regulations.

   c. identifies conditions that may lead to alleged malpractice.

   d. is unnecessary in an organized dental practice.

9. Major reason legal actions are decided in favor of the patient:

   a. A patient is right.

   b. The dentist is guilty.

   c. Dental assistant is unavailable to provide interpretation of clinical entries.

   d. Poor record keeping.

10. Characteristics of clinical record entries include all of the following EXCEPT

   a. signature, date, and identification number of person making the entry.

   b. use of standard abbreviations.

   c. consistent line spacing.

   d. marking an error and writing over.

11. Which is an example of an objective statement?

   a. Mrs. Oliver is in a strange mood today; she wants to be seen only by Dr. Edwards.

   b. Mrs. Oliver said, "I want to see only Dr. Edwards today."

COMPUTER APPLICATIONS EXERCISES

Preparing Clinical Records
Student Assignment #1
Go to the Evolve website and download the assignment for Chapter 8

Your assignment is to prepare a clinical record for four patients (information to follow). In each of the following chapters, you will be given an exercise that pertains to your patient and his or her clinical chart.

Step One: Create an electronic folder for each of the following four patients, Jana Rogers, Angelica Green, Holly Barry, and Lynn Bacca. Organize the folders in the *Clinical Records* folder located in your ADA WB.

Note: It is very important that you complete only the exercise assigned in each chapter.

Step Two: Create an electronic folder, name *Patient Forms* and place it in your *Clinical Records* folder located in your ADA WB. Download each of the electronic patient forms from the EVOLVE website and place them in the file you just created.

Step Three: Prepare clinical records for the following patients using the blank forms you just placed in the *Patient Forms* folder. Use the information given to complete the selected forms. Not all of the forms required for a clinical record will be included in the exercises. Where information is missing, leave the space blank.

Tip: After you open a blank form, rename the form using the patient's initials and the name of the form and place it in the patient's file. If you forget to do this, you will not have a blank form for your next patient; if this happens, go to the EVOLVE site and download a blank form.

1. Prepare a clinical record for Jana Rogers.

   Complete the following forms:

   - Registration Form

   - Clinical Examination Form

   - Treatment Plan Form

2. Prepare a clinical record for Angelica Green. Complete the following forms:

   - Registration Form

   - Medical and Dental Form

   - Clinical Examination Form

   - Periodontal Screening Form

   - Treatment Plan

3. Prepare a clinical record for Holly Barry. Select the forms you will need.

4. Prepare a clinical record for Lynn Bacca. Select the forms you will need.

Preparing Clinical Records

Your assignment is to prepare a clinical record for four patients (information to follow). In each of the following chapters, you will be given an exercise that pertains to your patient and his or her clinical chart.

Step One: Select a method by which to organize your patient's clinical record. The objective is to maintain a separate record for each patient. You will need one of the following:

- Four lateral file folders, four fasteners (you can also staple the records)
- Four horizontal file folders, four fasteners
- One three-ring notebook, four dividers

Note: It is very important that you complete only the exercise assigned in each chapter.

Step Two: Prepare clinical records for the following patients using the blank forms supplied in the appendix at the back of this workbook (p. 161). Use the information given to complete the selected forms. Not all of the forms required for a clinical record will be included in the exercises. Where information is missing, leave the space blank.

1. Prepare a clinical record for Jana Rogers.

   Complete the following forms:

   - Registration Form
   - Clinical Examination Form
   - Treatment Plan Form

2. Prepare a clinical record for Angelica Green. Complete the following forms:

   - Registration Form
   - Medical and Dental Form
   - Clinical Examination Form
   - Periodontal Screening Form
   - Treatment Plan

3. Prepare a clinical record for Holly Barry. Select the forms you will need.

4. Prepare a clinical record for Lynn Bacca. Select the forms you will need.

Patient Information

JANA J. ROGERS
Patient Information

Patient	Jana J. Rogers
Date of birth	3-12-2010
If child, parent name	Donald Rogers
How do you wish to be addressed	
Marital status	Single
Home address	8176 Hillside
City	Centerville
State/zip	NV 55555
Business address	
City	
State/zip	

Home phone.. 261-555-6217

Business phone..

Patient/parent employer... Valley Construction

Position... Foreman

How long.. 12 yrs

Spouse/parent name... Doris

Spouse employer.. Solutions Group

Position... N/A

How long..

Who is responsible for this account................................... Donald Rogers

Driver's license number.. C3261

Method of payment.. Insurance

Purpose of call.. Toothache

Other members in this practice... Donald, Doris, and Jason

Whom may we thank for this referral................................. Parents

Notify in case of emergency... Sadie Rogers
261-555-3001

Insurance Information 1st Coverage (Head of House)

Employee name... Donald Rogers

Employee date of birth.. 2/8/1969

Employer... Valley Construction

Name of insurance co... Prudential

Address... P.O. 15078
Albany, NY 12212-4094

Telephone.. 800-282-0555

Program or policy # 88442

Union local or group... VC

Social Security # 012-34-5678

Fee Schedule... None

Insurance Information 2nd coverage

Employee name... Doris Rogers

Employee date of birth.. 12/2/1972

Employer... Solutions Group

Name of insurance co... Principal Financial Group

Address... 10210 N 25th Ave, Phoenix, AZ 85021-3910

Telephone.. 800-328-8722

Program or policy # 88446

Union local or group... Solutions Group

Social Security # 632-24-7654

Fee Schedule... None

Provider... Dennis Smith Jr.

Privacy request... None

First visit... 4/12/

JANA J. ROGERS
Medical and Dental History Information

Medical information.. Normal (not necessary to complete for this exercise)

Allergies.. Penicillin

.... (enter in Med. Alert on all appropriate forms for this patient)

Dental Information... Normal (not necessary to complete for this exercise)

JANA J. ROGERS
Clinical Examination Information
Missing Teeth & Existing Restorations

2... MOD amalgam

13... O amalgam

14... B amalgam

18... DO composite

19... Sealant

30... MOD composite

1-16-17-32.. Extracted

Soft tissue examination okay

Oral hygiene fair

Calculus moderate

Gingival bleeding none

Perio exam no

Conditions/Treatment Indicated

3... DO composite/resin

15... OB composite/resin

18... B composite/resin

30... Apical abscess/root canal

30... Core build-up (pre-fab)

30... PFM (high noble) crown

JANA J. ROGERS
Treatment Plan

Date	Category	Tooth #	Procedure	Fee
4/12	Diagnostic		Examination	35.00
	Preventive		Prophy	60.00
	Diagnostic		4 bite-wing x-rays	40.00
	Diagnostic		1 PAs	16.00
5/17	Restorative	3	DO composite/resin	85.00
5/17	Restorative	15	OB composite/resin	85.00
4/24	Endodontic	30	Root canal	420.00
5/10	Endodontic	30	Post and core (pre-fab)	210.00
5/10	Restorative	30	PFM (high noble)	720.00
			Total Estimate	1671.00

All fees used in this exercise are for illustration only and do not represent actual fees charged for the procedures.

ANGELICA GREEN
Patient Information

Patient..	Angelica Green
Date of birth...	7/20/1992
If child, parent name...	
How do you wish to be addressed..	Angie
Marital status..	Married
Home address..	724 E. Mark Ave
City..	Northside
State/zip..	NV 22222
Business address...	3461 N. Cramer Ave
City..	Northside
State/zip..	NV 22222
Home phone...	801-555-3004
Business phone..	801-555-6134
Patient/parent employer..	James Taylor, DDS
Position..	RDA
How long...	4 yrs
Spouse/parent name..	Anthony Green
Spouse employer...	Pacific States
Position..	Accountant
How long...	8 yrs
Who is responsible for this account...	Anthony
Driver's license number...	60314
Method of payment..	Insurance
Purpose of call...	Toothache
Other members in this practice..	None
Whom may we thank for this referral...	Dr. Taylor
Patient/parent SS #	736-82-9176
Spouse/parent SS #	286-34-2212
Notify in case of emergency..	Grace Miller, 801-555-9909

Insurance Information 1st Coverage (Head of House)

Employee name..	Anthony Green
Employee date of birth...	9-13-1992
Employer..	Pacific States
Name of Insurance co...	Dental Select
Address...	5373 S Green St
....	Salt Lake City UT 84123-5432
Telephone...	800-999-9789
Program or policy #	95740
Union local or group..	Pacific States
Social Security #	286-34-2212
Fee Schedule..	None

63

Employee name...
Employee date of birth...
Employer...
Name of insurance co...
Address...
Telephone..
Program or policy # ....
Union local or group..
Social Security # ....
Provider.. Paula Pearson
Privacy request... No phone calls
First visit.. 3/6/

ANGELICA GREEN
Medical and Dental History Information

Medical information... Normal with following exceptions
Allergies.. Sulfa drugs and codeine (enter in Med. Alert on all
                                                                                                      appropriate forms for this patient)
                                                                                             Sensitive to latex
                                                                                             Bleeds easily when cut
Dental information.. Complete as much information as you can about the patient
Aware of problem.. Bleeding gums when I brush
Clench and grind teeth... Yes
Gums bleed.. Yes

ANGELICA GREEN
Clinical Examination Information
Missing Teeth & Existing Restoration

1.. Missing
2.. O composite
3.. B composite
14.. DO composite
16.. Missing
17.. Missing
32.. Missing

Chief Complaint: Bleeding Gums

Soft tissue examination... Normal
Oral hygiene.. Good
Calculus... Heavy
Gingival bleeding.. General
Perio exam... Yes

Conditions/Treatment Indicated

L/L	Periodontal scaling and root planing
U/L	Periodontal scaling and root planing
L/R	Periodontal scaling and root planing
U/R	Periodontal scaling and root planing

Periodontal Screening Examination

Tooth	Buccal	Lingual	Mobility	Furcation	Recession
2	676	455	1	2	1
3	876	767	1	2	1
4	444	444	0	0	0
14	876	765	1	2	1
15	453	543	1	2	1
18	547	665	1	1	0
19	767	878	1	1	0
30	455	445	1	1	0
31	667	778	1	1	0

ANGELICA GREEN
Treatment Plan

Date	Category	Tooth #	Procedure	Fee
3/6	Diagnostic		FMX	90.00
3/6	Diagnostic		Comprehensive exam	45.00
4/12	Perio	L/L	Periodontal scaling & root planing	175.00
4/12	Perio	U/L	Periodontal scaling & root planing	175.00
4/24	Perio	L/R	Periodontal scaling & root planing	175.00
4/24	Perio	U/R	Periodontal scaling & root planing	175.00
			Total Estimate	835.00

All fees used in this exercise are for illustration only and do not represent actual fees charged for the procedures.

HOLLY BARRY
Patient Information

Patient	Holly Barry
Date of birth	3/6/1942
If child, parent name	NA
How do you wish to be addressed	Mrs. Barry
Marital status	Widowed
Home address	3264 S. Vine St
City	Westside
State/zip	NV 44444
Business address	NA
City	
State/zip	

Home phone... 801-555-2331

Business phone... NA

Patient/parent employer.. NA

Position.. NA

How long.. NA

Spouse/parent name.. NA

Spouse employer.. NA

Position.. NA

How long.. NA

Who is responsible for this account.. Self

Driver's license number.. 36788

Method of payment... Credit Card

Purpose of call... New Denture

Other members in this practice... Son

.... Donald Rogers

Whom may we thank for this referral.. Donald

Patient/parent SS # 111-32-4356

Spouse/parent SS # .... NA

Notify in case of emergency.. Donald Rogers

Insurance Information 1st Coverage

Employee name... NA

Employee date of birth.. NA

Employer... NA

Name of insurance co. .... NA

Address... NA

Telephone... NA

Program or policy # .... NA

Union local or group.. NA

Social Security # .... NA

Insurance Information 2nd Coverage

Employee name... NA

Employee date of birth.. NA

Employer... NA

Name of insurance co. .... NA

Address... NA

Telephone... NA

Program or policy # .... NA

Union local or group.. NA

Social Security # .... NA

Provider.. Dennis Smith

Privacy request... none

First visit... 2/4

Fee Schedule.. None

HOLLY BARRY
Medical and Dental History Information

Medical information... Normal (not necessary to complete for this exercise)

Allergies... NONE (enter in Med. Alert on all appropriate forms for this patient)

SPECIAL NOTE... Patient cannot sit for long periods of time, must get out of the dental chair and stretch every 60 minutes

Dental information.. Normal (not necessary to complete for this exercise)

HOLLY BARRY
Clinical Examination Information
Missing Teeth & Existing Restorations

1-16... Missing

17-19... Missing

29.. MODLB Amalgam

U... Complete denture: Placed 1997, relined 3 times, loose fitting

L.. Partial denture: Placed 1992, broken clasp

Chief complaint: Lower right molar broken
Upper denture very loose

Soft Tissue Examination.. Normal

Oral Hygiene... Good

Calculus.. Moderate

Gingival Bleeding... None

Perio Exam... Yes

Conditions/Treatment Indicated

U... Complete denture

29.. PFM High noble

L.. Partial denture, metal clasp, and framework

HOLLY BARRY
Treatment Plan

Date	Category	Tooth #	Procedure	Fee
2/4	Diagnostic		FMX	90.00
2/4	Diagnostic		Examination (limited)	35.00
4/12	Restorative	29	PFM	650.00
	Prostho		Complete maxillary denture	950.00
4/30	Prostho		Mandibular partial denture	
			Cast metal framework	1,050.00
			Total Estimate	2775.00

All fees used in this exercise are for illustration only and do not represent actual fees charged for the procedures.

LYNN BACCA
Patient Information

Patient...	Lynn Bacca
Date of birth..	8/12/2016
If child, parent name...	Chuck Bacca
How do you wish to be addressed..	Lynn
Marital status...	Child
Home address...	1812 Harman Dr
City...	Southside
State/zip...	NV 33333
Business address..	34655 VIP Parkway
City...	Westside
State/zip...	NV 44444
Home phone...	801-555-3421
Business phone..	801-555-6210
Patient/parent employer..	Diamond Welding
Position..	Production Manager
How long..	8 yrs
Spouse/parent name...	Fern Bacca
Spouse employer..	Columbia Healthcare
Position..	Speech Pathologist
How long..	5 yrs
Who is responsible for this account...	Father
Driver's license number...	878765
Method of payment...	Insurance
Purpose of call...	Exam
Other members in this practice..	Parents, brother Steve
Whom may we thank for this referral...	Aunt, Evelyn Evatt 3245 S. Spring St Canyon View, CA 91711
Notify in case of emergency..	Parent

Insurance Information 1st Coverage

Employee name..	Chuck Bacca
Employee date of birth...	7/27/1987
Employer..	Diamond Welding
Name of insurance co.	Delta Dental Plan
Address...	PO 7736 San Francisco CA 94120
Telephone...	415-972-8300
Program or policy #	12121
Union local or group..	Diamond
Social Security #	026-81-9217
Fee Schedule..	None

Employee name.. Fern Bacca
Employee date of birth... 7/5/1990
Employer... Columbia Healthcare
Name of insurance co. .... Connecticut General
Address... PO 1650
Visalia, CA 93279

Telephone.. 800-252-2091
Program or policy # 55001
Union local or group .... Columbia
Social Security # 213-90-7148
Fee Schedule... None
Provider... Brenda Childs
Privacy request.. None
First visit... 4/12

LYNN BACCA
Medical and Dental History Information

Medical information... Normal (not necessary to complete for this exercise)
Allergies.. (enter in Med. Alert on all appropriate forms for this patient)
Dental information.. Normal (not necessary to complete for this exercise)

LYNN BACCA
Clinical Examination Information
Missing Teeth and Existing Restorations

No Existing Restorations or Missing Teeth
Soft tissue examination... Normal
Oral hygiene.. Good
Calculus.. None
Gingival bleeding... None
Perio exam... No

Conditions/Treatment Indicated

3...	Sealant
14...	Sealant
19...	Sealant
30...	Sealant

LYNN BACCA
Treatment Plan

Date	Category	Tooth #	Procedure	Fee
4/12	Diagnostic		BW x-Rays (4)	40.00
	Diagnostic		2 ANT PA's	14.00
	Preventive		Prophy and Fluoride TX	54.00
4/24	Preventive	3	Sealant	32.00
	Preventive	14	Sealant	32.00

Preventive	19	Sealant.. 32.00
Preventive	30	Sealant.. 32.00
		Total Estimate.. 236.00

All fees used in this exercise are for illustration only and do not represent actual fees charged for the procedures.

Practice Management Software Exercise
Student Assignment # 2 (Option 1).
If you have access to a practice management software system other than Dentrix, your assignment is to prepare electronic clinical records for four patients (information given on the previous pages). In each of the following chapters, you will be given an exercise that pertains to your patient and his or her electronic clinical record. <u>Please note</u>: Step-by-step instruction will not be given if this option is chosen. Your instructor will be able to provide the instruction you may need to complete these assignments.

Tip: Some software programs will not allow you to use addresses and zip codes that are fictitious. If you encounter this problem, please make changes following your instructor's guidance.

Complete the following tasks:

1. Create an electronic clinical record for Jana J. Rogers and enter the following information.

   - Registration information

   - Clinical Examination information

   - Treatment Plan information

2. Create an electronic clinical record for Angelica Green and enter the following information.

   - Registration information

   - Medical and Dental History

   - Clinical Examination Information

   - Periodontal Screening Information

   - Treatment Plan

3. Create an electronic clinical record for Holly Barry. Select the information you will need.

4. Create an electronic clinical record for Lynn Bacca. Select the information you will need.

Dentrix Learning Edition Lessons
Student Assignment #2 (option 2)
Go to the Evolve website and complete the Dentrix Learning Edition Lesson assignments for Chapter 8.
Lesson: Patient Records
   Creating a New Family Record
   Adding a Family Member to a Family Record
   Assigning a Billing Type to a Patient
   Changing the Head of House for a Family
   Assigning Items to a Patient's Health History

DENTRIX APPLICATION EXERCISES

Dentrix Student Learning Outcomes
The student will:

- Create a Family File for new patients and their families.

- Enter important patient information, such as patient demographics, medical alerts, and employer and insurance information.

- Create and print a pretreatment plan.

User's Guide Resources

Chapter 3: Family File

    Adding a New Family (Account)

    Adding Family Members

    Assigning Medical Conditions

    Assigning Employers

    Insurance

Chapter 7: Treatment Planner

    Opening the Treatment Planner

    Creating Treatment Plan Cases

Chapter 8: Ledger

    Ledger Overview

Dentrix Guided Practice

Creating a family file

To add a new family into the Learning Edition, you must create a file for the head-of-house. Once the head-of-house has been entered, you can add each additional family member to the family. *Note:* If the head-of-house is not a patient, change the status from *patient* to *nonpatient* (located in the drop-down menu in the *Status* field). For detailed information on how to complete the Head-of-House Information box, refer to the Dentrix *User's Guide,* Family File-Adding a New Family (Account).

    To create a file for the head-of-house:

1. In the Family File, click the **Select Patient/New Family** button. The Select Patient dialogue box appears.

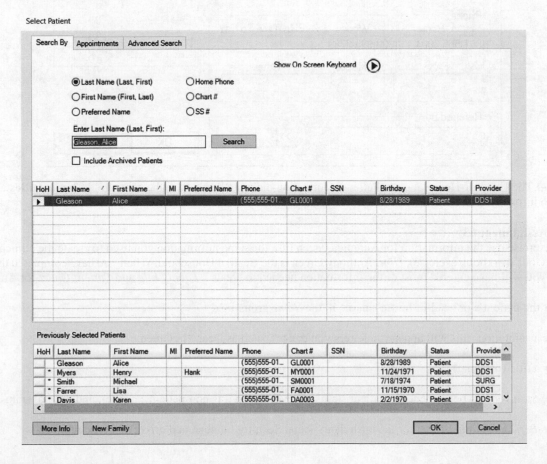

2. Click **New Family**. The Head-of House Information dialogue box appears.

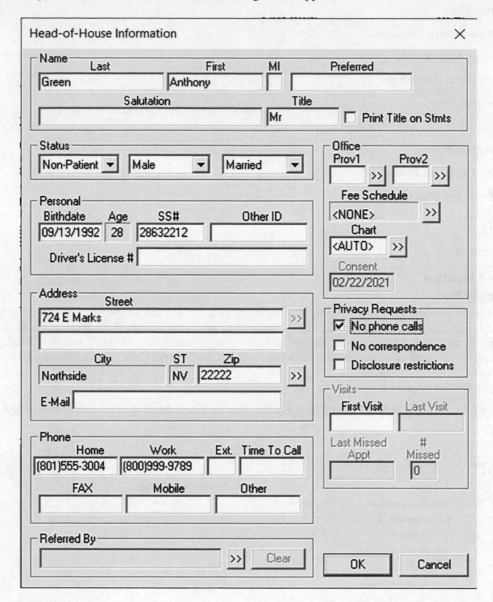

(*Note:* The Head-of-House and the Patient Information dialogue boxes have the same fields, but the titles are different to inform you to enter the head-of-house's or new family member's information.)

Student Assignment #3

For this exercise use the information for Angelica Green (use the same information you used to create the clinical records in the previous workbook exercise). *Hint:* Anthony Green is the Head of Household. When you have completed the guided practice, you will have entered most of the information needed to create a *Family File* and *Patient Chart* for Angelica.

3. Enter the patient's or head-of house's name in the *Name* group box.

4. Enter a salutation (this will appear on letters you create), such as Dear Mr. Green.

5. Enter a title (optional).

6. In the *Status group* box, select the patient status (for Mr. Green it is non-patient), gender, and marital status.

7. In the *Personal group* box, enter the birth date, Social Security number, and driver's license number.

8. In the *Other* field in the Personal group box is used on some insurance forms when a separate patient ID is required to file a claim.

9. In the *Address* group box, enter the street address, zip code, and e-mail address in the corresponding fields.

10. In the *Office* group box, select the primary and secondary providers (DDS1).

11. Select the option in the *Privacy Request* group box, if applicable.

12. Click **OK** to save and add the head-of-house to the database.

Adding Family Members

Follow these steps after you have entered all the information related to the head-of-house:

1. Click the **Add Family Member** button on the toolbar. The Patient Information dialogue box appears. The last name, provider, home phone number, and address default to the information entered for the head-of-house file.

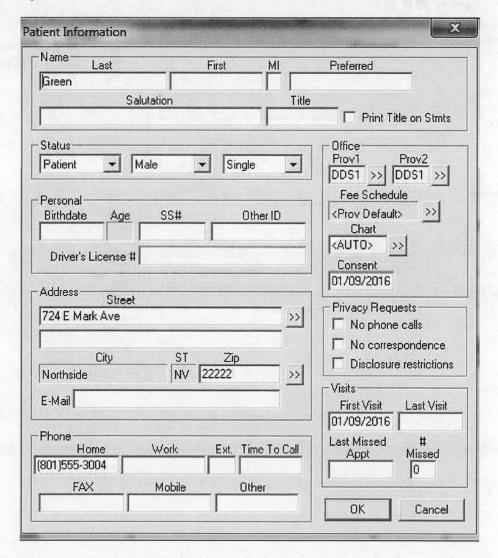

2. Enter Family member information (Angelica Green) in the appropriate field. Hint: Check Angelica's information carefully, she has a different provider and privacy request.

3. Click OK.

Note: Refer to the Dentrix User's Guide Family File – Adding a new Family section for a complete explanation of each field.

Assigning Medical Conditions to Patient

Once you have created a file for a patient in the Family File, you may need to add medical conditions to the patient. To add medical conditions to a patient:

1. In the Family File, select a patient (Angelica Green).

2. Double click the **Health History** block. Health History appears.

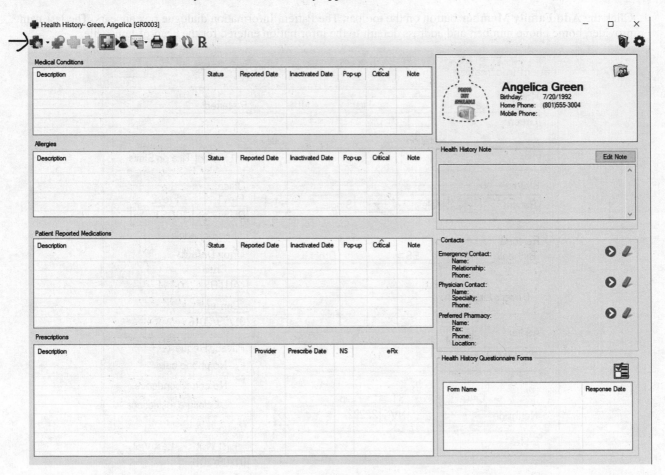

3. Click the Add toolbar button, and then click Add Multiple. The Add Multiple dialog box appears.

Health History - Add Multiple for Green, Angelica

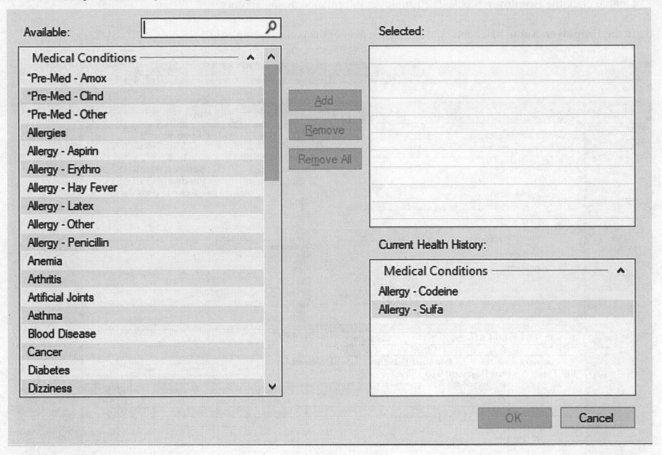

4. Select the appropriate conditions from the list, and then click **Add** to move them to the list.

5. Click **OK** to return to the Health History.

6. Click the Family File button to return to the Health History dialog box.

7. Click **OK**.

Assigning an Employer to the Patient

1. In the Family File, select a patient (Angelica Green).

2. Double click the **Employer** Block. The Employer Information dialog appears.

3. In the **Employer Name** field, enter the first few letters of the patient's employer.

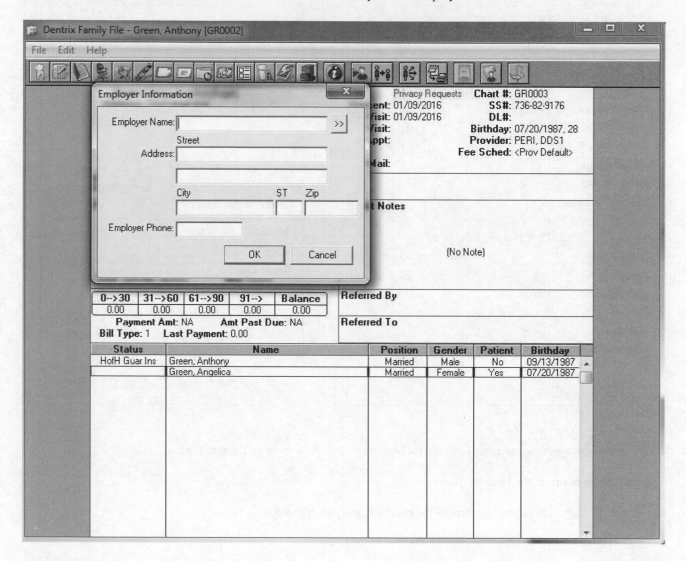

4. Click the **Employer Name** search button to determine whether the employer is already in the database to help avoid duplicates. The Select Employer dialog appears.

5. Select the employer or enter the employer's information. Note: If the employer's information is not listed, click **Cancel** to return to the Employer Information dialog and complete the fields.

6. Click **OK** to return to the Family File.

Assigning Insurance

Note: To assign insurance to a patient, the insurance subscriber must be listed as a family member in the patient's Family File. If the subscriber is not a patient, set the status to *Nonpatient* in the subscriber's patient information and complete the insurance information.

Assigning Primary Insurance to a Subscriber

1. From the Family File, select the patient/subscriber (Anthony Green).

2. Double click the **Insurance Information** block. The Insurance Information dialogue box appears. Select the subscriber of the insurance (Anthony Green).

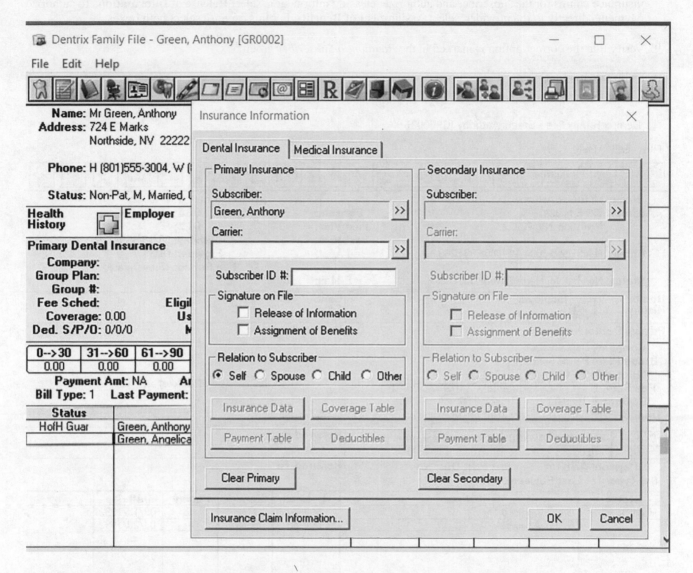

3. Click the **Carrier** search button. (≫) The Select Primary Dental Insurance Plan dialog appears.

4. In the *Search By* group box, mark the desired search method.

5. Enter the first few letters/numbers of the selected search method in the field provided.

6. Select the desired plan. If the plan is not listed, follow the steps outlined in the *Entering a New Insurance Plan* in the *User's Guide*. If the plan is listed, select the plan from the list and click **OK** to return to the Insurance Information dialog box.

7. Verify that the subscriber ID number is correct (add the information if missing). The subscriber ID may be the Social Security number of the subscriber. However, because of HIPAA regulations, you can use a number other than the subscriber's Social Security number.

8. Verify that the correct options are checked in the *Signature on File* group box. To print "Signature on File" on the insurance claims for the subscriber and authorize releasing information, select **Release of Information**. To authorize payments directly to the provider, select **Assignment of Benefits**. For this exercise select both boxes.

9. Verify that the correct option is marked in the *Relation to Subscriber* group box.

10. Click **OK** to return to the Family File.

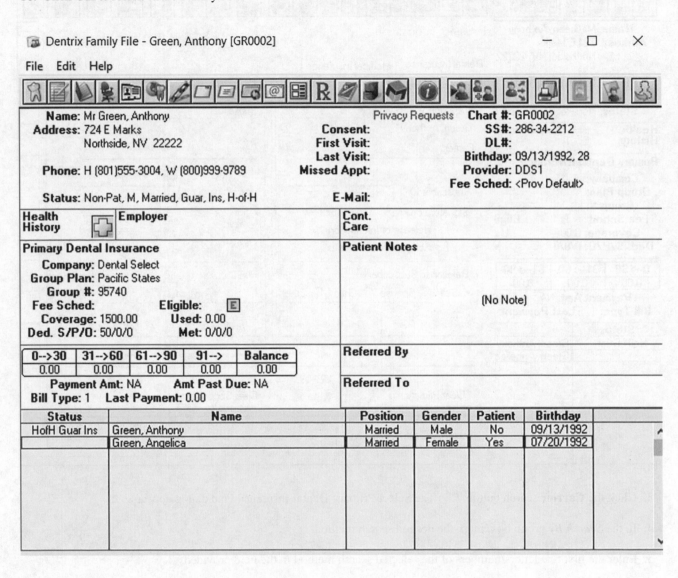

Assigning Primary Insurance to a Patient (non-subscriber)

1. From the Family File, select the patient (Angelica Green).

2. Double click the **Insurance Information** block. The Insurance Information dialogue box appears.

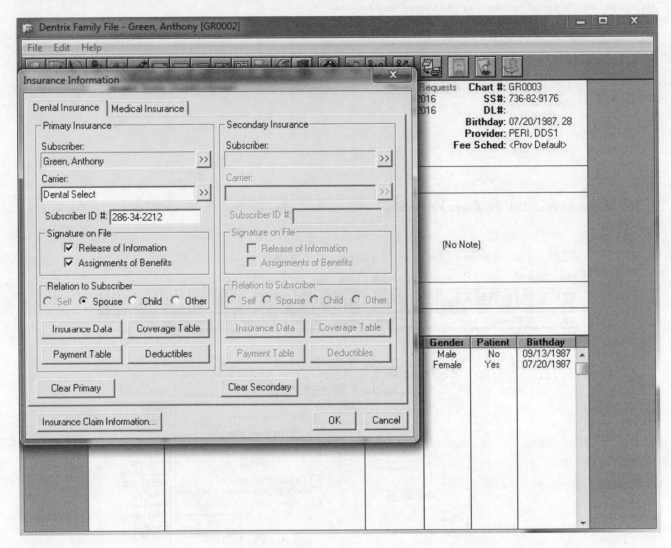

3. Click the **Search** button (≫) next to **Subscriber.** The Select Primary Subscriber dialogue box appears.

4. Select the primary subscriber and click **OK** to return to the Insurance Information dialogue box. *Note:* If the subscriber is not listed, you will need to add him or her as a patient and assign insurance information before you can continue.

5. Select Release of Information and Assignments of Benefits.

6. Select Self, Spouse, Child, or Other as the patient's relation to the subscriber.

7. If the patient has secondary insurance coverage, enter the information in the *Secondary Insurance* box.

8. Click **OK** to return to the Family File.

Creating a Treatment Plan Case

1. Click the **Select Patient** button on the Ledger toolbar. Enter the first few letters of the patient's last name (Angelica Green). Select the desired patient and click **OK.** *Note:* If you have the patient's file open in Family File, select the Ledger button from the toolbar; this will open the patient's ledger.

79

2. From the Ledger menu bar, select Options, then Treatment Plan. *Note:* The Ledger Title Bar now reflects that you are in the Treatment Plan View.

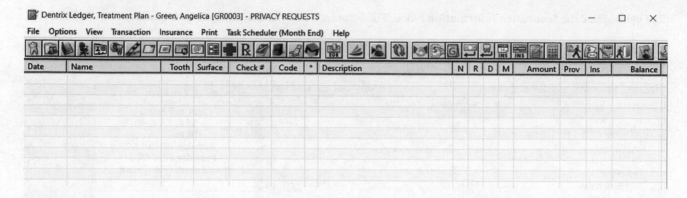

3. To add procedures, click the **Enter Procedure** button on the Ledger toolbar. The Enter Procedure(s) dialogue box appears.

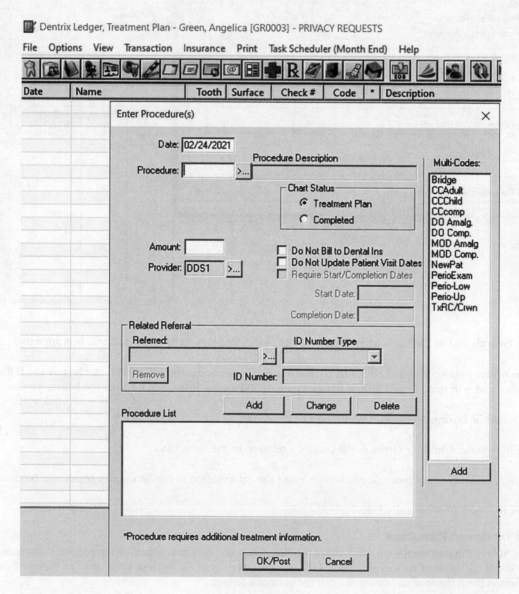

Add procedures to the Procedure list using individual codes or selecting the search button. Select the appropriate ADA Category. All procedure codes assigned to that category are displayed in the Procedure List. Select the desired code and click **OK.**

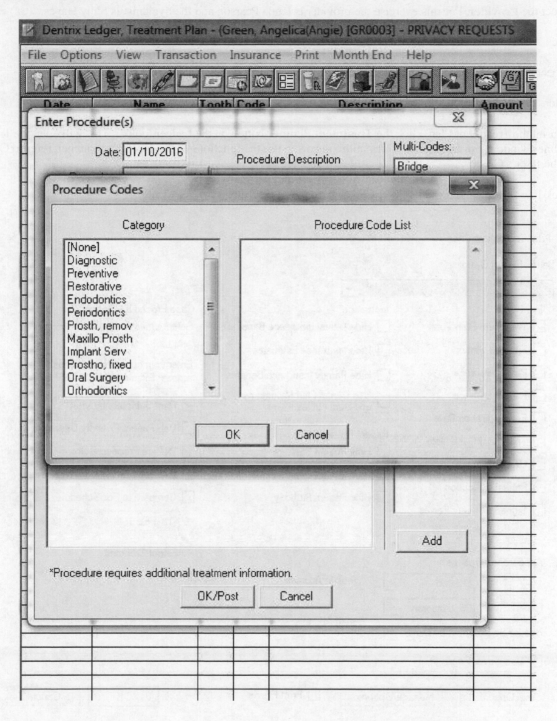

4. If the procedure code requires additional treatment information such as surface, tooth number, or quadrant, you should enter those now.

5. Chart Status select Treatment Plan.

6. Once a procedure code has been selected, a fee will be automatically assigned according to the fee schedule on file. However, you can enter a different fee in the **Amount** field. Use the fees listed on Angelica's worksheet.

7. Select the **Provider.** For this exercise the provider is Paula Pearson and the hygienist is Sally Hayes.

8. Click **Add** to add this procedure to the Procedure Pane.

9. Repeat steps 1 through 8 for all procedures.

10. When all procedures have been listed, click **OK/POST.**

11. To print the Treatment Plan, click the **Treatment Planner** button on the Ledger toolbar. This will open the Treatment Planner window. For additional information on how to use the functions of the Treatment Planner, refer to Chapter 7 in the User's Guide.

12. Click File > Print > Treatment Case. Check Treatment Plan Total Case.

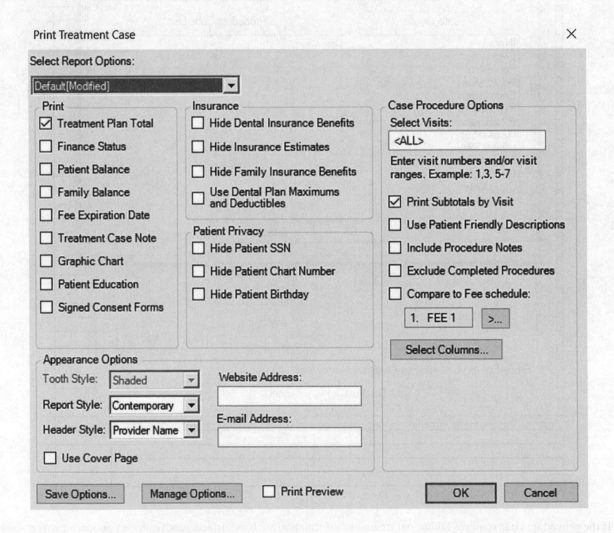

Dentrix Independent Practice

For this exercise you will use the same information you used to create clinical records for Jana Rogers, Angelica Green, Holly Barry, and Lynn Bacca.

1. Prepare a Family File for the Rogers family.

   A. Create a New Family with Donald Rogers as head-of-house.

   Note: Assign subscriber insurance information by double clicking on the Insurance Information Block (see directions above).

   B. Add Doris as a new family member (see directions above to assign subscriber insurance information).

   C. Add Jana as a new family member (see directions above to assign insurance).

   D. Create a pretreatment estimate for Jana (see directions above).

2. Prepare a Family File for the Green family. You have completed the majority of this assignment during the Dentrix Practice exercise. Review the file and check for completeness.

   A. Create a New Family with Anthony Green as H/H. (*Note:* Anthony is not a patient.) Assign subscriber insurance information.

   B. Add Angelica as a new family member and assign insurance.

   C. Create a pretreatment estimate for Angelica.

3. Prepare a Family File for Holly Barry.

   A. Create a New Family with Holly as H/H and patient.

   B. Create a pretreatment estimate for Holly.

4. Prepare a Family File for the Bacca family.

   A. Create a New Family with Chuck as H/H. Assign subscriber insurance information.

   B. Add Fern as a new family member and assign subscriber insurance information.

   C. Add Lynn as a new family member.

5. Check the total estimate for each patient on the worksheet in the workbook. Do the figures match the total estimate on the patient's treatment plan? (*Hint:* If the totals do not match, did you change the fee when entering the procedure information?) Correct any figures that are not correct.

6. Print out a copy of each patient's treatment plan (Jana, Angelica, and Holly) and place in the patient's clinical record.

Dentrix Charting

If you completed the charting exercises in Chapter 2 and would like additional practice charting, use the Patient Chart module to enter the treatment for the above patients. Use the information provided in the Clinical Exam Information and Treatment Plan for each patient (information was provided earlier in this chapter of the workbook.)

Continue working on your Dental Practice Procedural Manual (see Workbook Chapter 6 for details).
   Suggested activities:

■ Team meeting

■ Review timeline

■ Review Group research and writing assignments

■ Complete research and writing assignments for this chapter

■ Review and revise completed sections of the manual

■ Individual journal entries

Information Management and Security

LEARNING OBJECTIVES

1. Discuss and give examples of security risks for different types of EHR hosts.
2. List and describe the 10 tips for cybersecurity in health care.
3. List and describe the six filing methods outlined in this chapter, including demonstration of the ARMA Simplified Filing Standard Rules.
4. Compare and contrast the filing methods used for business records such as accounts payable and personnel records versus patient and insurance information.
5. Prepare a new patient's clinical record for filing.
6. Prepare a business document for filing (manually and electronically).
7. Discuss how long records must be retained and the two methods of transferring records.

INTRODUCTION

The responsibilities of the administrative dental assistant in the management and security of information and records are multifaceted. In today's dental practice, the storage of information may involve both paper files and electronic files. Although methods of documentation may vary, the principles of a records management program will always be the same. According to the International Organization for Standardization (ISO), in *Information and Documentation-Records Management,* a general policy should involve "… the creation and management of authentic, reliable and useable records, capable of supporting business function and activities for as long as they are required." In addition to the management of the information it is also necessary to ensure that the information is safe from loss or unauthorized access. Federal HIPAA rules and state mandates have specific laws and regulations to ensure PHI is protected. The importance of collecting the correct information and preparation of a dental record was discussed in Chapter 8. This chapter discusses key elements of the HIPAA Rules and basic methods used in a systematic approach to the storage and retrieval of information (filing).

EXERCISES

1. What criteria must be maintained once a clinical record has been created?

   _____

   _____

   _____

   _____

2. Check all of the following that may be considered a business associate.

   Cleaning service _____

   Billing service _____

   Insurance billing service _____

   Dental technician _____

   Dental assisting intern _____

Bank manager _____

Practice management software technician _____

Insurance clearinghouse _____

Dental supply representative _____

3. What does the Privacy Rule protect?

_____

_____

_____

4. True or False: The Privacy Rule only applies to PHI in a EHR.

5. What does the Security Rule establish?

_____

_____

_____

6. List and describe the three safeguards outlined in the Security Rule.

a. _____

_____

_____

_____

b. _____

_____

_____

_____

c. _____

_____

_____

_____

7. What is cybersecurity and why is it important in a dental practice?

_____

_____

_____

_____

8. What is the main purpose of managing documents and information in a dental practice?

_____

_____

_____

9. List the six basic filing methods and give an example of how they may be used in a dental practice.

_____

_____

_____

10. Explain the order in which electronic records are organized.

_____

_____

_____

_____

11. Using the personal name rule, identify which information will be placed in the following:

Unit 1 _____

Unit 2 _____

Unit 3 _____

Unit 4 _____

12. Using the business rule, identify which information will be placed in the following:

Unit 1_____

Unit 2_____

Unit 3_____

Unit 4_____

13. When a numeric filing system is used for patient records, a key component in locating the record is

    a. charts are arranged numerically.

    b. charts are color-coded.

    c. charts are randomly assigned numbers.

    d. charts are cross-referenced.

14. Geographic category records are filed according to

    a. ZIP code.

    b. area code.

    c. city.

    d. state.

    e. all of the above.

15. Subject filing is a method of filing strictly by subject. True or false, and why?

_____

_____

_____

16. Which method indexes by date?

_____

17. **Matching:** Identify the method of filing that would be used when a system is established for the following types of business documents. If a system uses two methods, list the primary location first and the secondary method second. For example: Personnel files are first filed by subject (S) (primary location) and then filed alphabetically (A) by employee (secondary method). The answer will be S/A.

a. ___/___Accounts payable   S. Subject

b. ___/___Accounts receivable (ledger)   G. Geographic

c. ___/___Bank statements   A. Alphabetical

d. ___/___Financial reports   N. Numerical

e. ___/___Personnel records   C. Chronological

f. ___/___Payroll records

g. ___/___Tax records

h. ___/___Business reports

i. ___/___Insurance reports (business)

j. ___/___Insurance claims (patient)

k. ___/___Professional correspondence

l. ___/___Patient information.

18. Maintaining an active filing system requires the removal of inactive records and documents. Identify two types of transfer methods and briefly describe how each method works.

_____

_____

_____

_____

_____

_____

_____

_____

_____

_____

_____

_____

_____

COMPUTER APPLICATION EXERCISE

Go to the Evolve website and download the assignment for Chapter 9.

Student Assignment #1

1. Complete the assignment.

2. Print a copy of the completed assignment and place an electronic copy in your ADA WB Chapter 9 folder.

Student Assignment #2

In the previous chapters you have created an electronic filing system through various computer applications assignments. For this chapter's assignment you will evaluate the organization and effectiveness of your electronic filing system and make adjustments if needed. Write you report and place it in your ADA WB Chapter 9 folder. Hint: you may want to take a before and after screen shot of your electronic filing system.

ACTIVITY EXERCISE (COMPLETE IF YOU HAVE CREATED PAPER FILES IN CHAPTER 8)

Complete the preparation of clinical records by preparing a file label for the following patients:

Jana Rogers

Angelica Green

Holly Barry

Lynn Bacca

WHAT WOULD YOU DO?

You have been asked to write the new office policy for safeguarding patients' clinical records (paper or electronic, your choice). You will need to research HIPAA policy and procedures. How will this be applied to a dental office?

1. Identify the type of records you will be addressing in your procedure guide (electronic or paper).

2. Research the HIPAA Policy for your selected choice.

3. Write a HIPAA Procedures Guide to be used in a dental office.

DENTAL PRACTICE PROCEDURAL MANUAL PROJECT (OPTIONAL)

Continue working on your Dental Practice Procedural Manual (see Workbook Chapter 6 for details).
   Suggested activities:

- Team meeting
- Review timeline
- Review Group research and writing assignments
- Complete research and writing assignments for this chapter
- Review and revise completed sections of the manual
- Individual journal entries

10 Dental Patient Scheduling

LEARNING OBJECTIVES

1. Describe the mechanics of scheduling, including the criteria required for matrixing an appointment book.
2. Discuss the art of scheduling and how to maximize scheduling efficiency, including the different methods used to identify when specific procedures should be scheduled.
3. Explain the seven different scenarios of appointment scheduling and formulate an action plan to solve the problems.
4. Describe the four ways that patients may schedule an appointment, including the use of traditional and alternative types of appointment cards and reminders.
5. Explain how use of a call list and daily schedule sheets can save time in the dental office.
6. List the steps to be followed in performing the daily routine associated with the appointment schedule.

INTRODUCTION

Developing and implementing an organized, functional schedule for a dental practice requires time, experience, and the cooperation of the entire dental healthcare team. The process of scheduling appointments involves more than entering names in a book or keying into a computer. Scheduling is a complex process that has two main elements. The first is the **mechanics of scheduling**, which includes selecting the appointment book (manual or electronic), outlining or **matrixing**, and entering information.

The second is the **"art" of scheduling**. The art of scheduling begins with the dental healthcare team and answering a few critical questions. These questions focus on the amount of time that is needed to complete procedures and take into consideration the total time the patient is in the chair. This will include how much time is needed by each individual team member during the patient's visit. The second step is to develop a process for monitoring and adjusting the schedule to meet the financial goals set by the dental healthcare team.

EXERCISES

1. A column in an appointment book is assigned to

    a. an individual practitioner.

    b. a treatment room.

    c. be used for information.

    d. all of the above.

2. If an appointment book has four time slots per hour, each time slot represents _____.

    a. 10 minutes

    b. 15 minutes

    c. 20 minutes

    d. 30 minutes

3. The dentist tells you that Judy will need 9 units for her next appointment (you are scheduling at 10-minute intervals). How long will Judy's appointment be?

    a. 1 hour

    b. 1 hour 10 minutes

    c. 1 hour 20 minutes

    d. 1 hour 30 minutes

4. What are the key questions that should be addressed by the dental healthcare team to increase productivity through effective scheduling?

_____

_____

_____

_____

5. Place the following tasks in order. Place the number 1 in front of the first task to be completed, 2 before the second, and so on.

a. _____ Check patients' charts for any information that may not have been included on the schedule, such as need for premedication, payments due, or updated insurance and medical information.

b. _____ Confirm or remind patients of their upcoming appointments.

c. _____ Confirm the return of laboratory work.

d. _____ Give the patient list to the dental assisting staff to review before they see the patients.

e. _____ Keep the dental healthcare team and patients informed of any changes that will affect their schedules.

f. _____ Pull the patients' clinical records, and review the procedures that are going to be completed the following day.

g. _____ Spend 5 to 10 minutes with the dental healthcare team to review the daily schedule.

h. _____ Print the daily schedule.

i. _____ Update schedules throughout the day as changes occur.

j. _____ Use the call list to fill any openings in the day's schedule.

COMPUTER APPLICATION EXERCISE

Student Assignment #1

Go to the Evolve website and download the assignment for Chapter 10.

1. Complete the assignment.

2. Print a copy of the completed assignment and place an electronic copy in your ADA WB Chapter 10 folder.

Dentrix Learning Edition Lessons
Student Assignment #2

Go to the Evolve website and complete the Dentrix Learning Edition Lesson assignments for Chapter 10.
Lesson: Scheduling
    Getting Started With the Appointment Book
    Identifying Appointment Book Symbols
    Identifying Areas of the Appointment Book
    Scheduling an Appointment for an Existing Patient

DENTRIX APPLICATION EXERCISES

Dentrix Student Learning Outcomes

The student will:

- Set up the practice schedule.

- Determine available appointment times.

- Schedule appointments for patients.

Dentrix User's Guide Resources

Chapter 4: Appointment Book

- The Appointment Book Window

- Finding Open Appointment Times

- Scheduling Appointments

- Changing Schedule Hours

DENTRIX GUIDED PRACTICE

The Dentrix Appointment Book (or any electronic scheduler) is an essential component of the practice management software program. The electronic appointment book allows you to track appointments; color code providers, procedures, and operatories; print route slips; and communicate vital patient information.

Operatory Setup

Before you begin, it will be necessary to determine the number of operatories that will be included in your appointment book. For this exercise you will be using five new operatories.

Student Assignment #3

1. In the Office Manager, select **Maintenance-Practice Setup-Practice Resource Setup**. The Practice Resource Setup dialogue box appears.

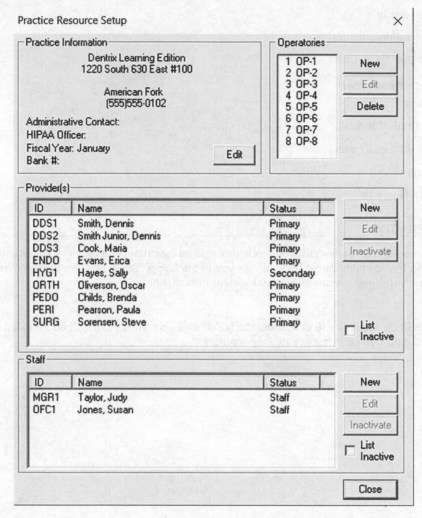

2. In the Operatories group box, Click **New** to add a new operatory. In the Operatory Information box assign a 4-digit ID, click **OK**. For this exercise you will add a total of five new operatories using the following IDs: ADA1, ADA2, ADA3, ADA4, and ADA5.

3. Click **Close.**

Setting Up the Appointment Book

The **Practice Appointment Setup** options in Appointment Book allow you to customize your practice hours, some appointment defaults, and the time block size.

    To set up practice hours:

Student Assignment #4

1. In Appointment Book, from the **Setup** menu, click **Practice Appointment Setup.** The **Practice Appointment Setup** dialogue box appears used.

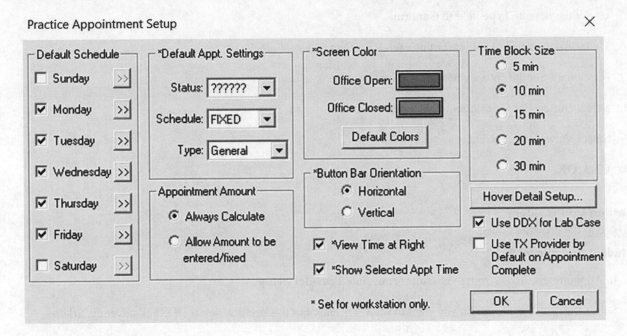

2. Dentrix allows you to schedule your appointments in 5-minute, 10-minute, 15-minute, 20-minute, or 30-minue intervals. Click the **Time Block Size.** (*Note:* In this exercise it will be a 10-minute interval.)

3. Dentrix defaults to a Monday through Friday workweek.

   a. Select the days of the week the office is usually open. (*Note:* For this exercise the office is open Monday through Friday.)

   b. Clear the days the office is closed.

4. You can set working hours for each selected day.

   a. Click the **search** button (≫) to the right of the day.

   b. To change the time range for a time block, click the Start Time or End Time **Search** button (≫) of the time block you want to change.

   Note: For this exercise, set the following times:

Monday	8:00 AM to 12:00 PM and 1:00 PM to 5:00 PM
Tuesday	8:00 AM to 12:00 PM and 1:30 PM to 5:30 PM
Wednesday	10:00 AM to 2:00 PM and 2:30 pm to 8:00 PM
Thursday	10:00 AM to 2:00 PM and 2:30 PM to 8:00 PM
Friday	10:00 AM to 1:00 PM and 1:20 PM to 3:00 PM

   c. When finished click **OK.**

5. Specify the default settings you want the Appointment Book to use for each new appointment when it is created.

   a. Set the default **Status** field to **??????.**

   b. Set the default **Schedule** field to **Fixed.**

   c. Set the default **Type** field to **General.**

6. Under Appointment Amount for this exercise, select Always Calculate.

7. (Optional). Set the colors you want Appointment Book to display.

8. Select Button Bar Orientation, Horizontal or Vertical.

9. Select View Time at Right.

10. Click **OK.**

Setting Up Providers

To set up the provider hours:

Student Assignment #5

1. In Appointment Book, from the **Setup** menu, click **Provider Setup.**

2. Select the provider for whom you want to set a schedule. For this exercise select DDS1 (Dr. Dennis Smith).

3. Click **Setup**.

   The **Provider Setup** dialogue box appears.

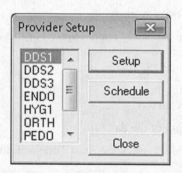

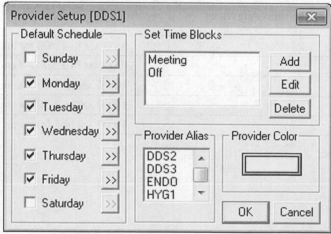

4. Select the days of the week the provider usually works.

5. Set the working hours for each selected day.

   You can set working hours for each selected day.

   a. Click the **search** button (≫) to the right of the day.

   b. To change the time range for a time block, click the Start Time or End Time **Search** button (≫) of the time block you want to change.

      Note: For this exercise, set the following times:

Monday	8:00 am-12:00 pm and 1:00 pm-5:00 pm
Tuesday	8:00 am-12:00 pm and 1:30 pm to 5:30 pm
Wednesday	10:00 am-2:00 pm and 2:30 pm to 8:00 pm
Thursday	10:00 am-2:00 pm and 2:30 pm to 8:00 pm
Friday	10:00 am-1:00 pm and 1:20 pm to 3:00 pm

   c. When finished click **OK**.

6. If desired, edit the provider's appointment book color in the Provider Color group box by clicking the color button.

7. Click **OK** to save changes.

8. Click **Close** to return to the Appointment Book.

   Repeat this process to setup the following providers:

   DDS2 (Dr. Dennis Smith, Jr.)

   PEDO (Dr. Brenda Childs)

   HYG1 (Sally Hayes)

Scheduling Appointments

Scheduling appointments can be done in several different ways depending on the type and complexity of the appointment (for a full description refer to the Dentrix User's Guide).

Student Assignment #6

Scheduling (quick start)

The following instructions explain the simplest way to schedule an appointment.

1. Either by manually finding an appointment time or by using the Dentrix Find feature (discussed in the Dentrix *User's Guide*), locate and open schedule space.

2. In the Appointment Book, double click the appropriate operatory at the time you want to schedule the appointment. For this exercise schedule the appointment for next Monday at 10 am in operatory ADA3. The **Select Patient** dialogue box appears.

3. Enter the first few letters of the patient's last name (Green).

4. Select the patient you want from the list (Angelica Green), and then click **OK.** The **Appointment Information** dialogue box appears. The **Provider** field defaults to the patient's primary provider.

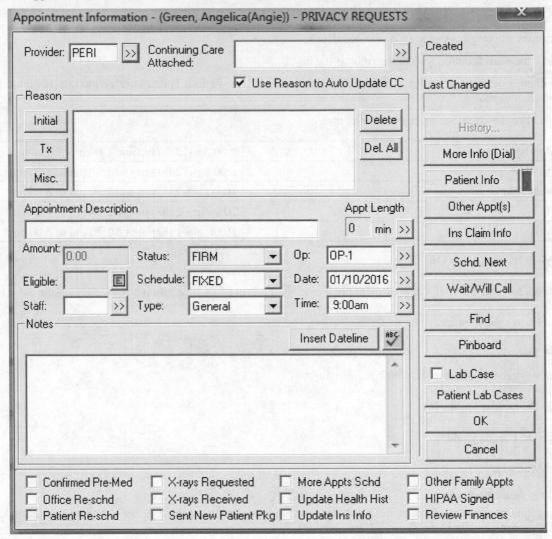

5. If necessary, click the **Provider** search button (≫) to select another provider for the appointment. (Select HYG1 as the provider.)

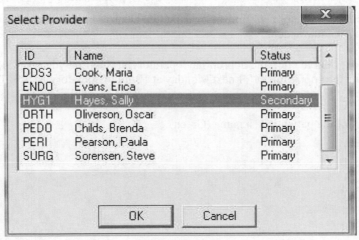

6. Under **Reason,** select a reason for the appointment using any of the following methods:

   a. If you are seeing the patient for a treatment that was previously planned, click **Tx.** In the **Treatment Plan** dialogue box, select the reasons for the appointment (comprehensive examination and FMX), and then click **Close.** *Note:* For this exercise click No in response to the Dentrix Continuing Care message.

   b. If you are seeing the patient for work that would be done on an initial visit, such as an exam or a cleaning, click **Initial.** In the **Select Initial Reasons** dialogue box, select the reasons for the appointment and then click **OK.**

   c. To add a new treatment-planned procedure, click **New Tx.** In the **Enter Procedure(s)** dialogue box, click the **Procedure** search button (≫), select the procedures you want from the **Procedure Codes** dialogue box, and then click **OK.** In the **Enter Procedure(s)** dialogue box, click **OK/Post.** In the **Treatment Plan** dialogue box, select the procedure you want for the appointment and click **Close.**

   d. If you are seeing the patient for a treatment that has not been planned, click **Misc.** In the **Procedure Codes** dialogue box, select a **Category** from the list; under **Procedure Code List,** select the procedure code you want, and then click **OK.**

7. Once you have entered a reason, Dentrix automatically assigns a length of time to the appointment.

   a. To change the length, click the **Appt Length** search button ≫.

   b. In the **Appointment Time Pattern** dialogue box, click the right arrow to increase or the left arrow to decrease the number of minutes needed, and then click **OK.**

8. Click **OK** to save any changes you have made and close the **Appointment Information** dialogue box.

Practice Management Software Exercise

Option 1. If you have access to a practice management software system other than Dentrix, your assignment is to schedule your patients (Jana, Angelica, Holly, and Lynn). Before you begin, you will need to be familiar with the electronic appointment book. The appointment book should be matrixed, and you have decided whether you will be assigning an operatory to a specific provider. For example, does the hygienist work out of one room? Are there specific operatories assigned to the different providers? For this exercise all your patients should be scheduled on the same day.

1. Jana Rogers (1 hour)

   a. Examination

   b. Prophy

   c. 4-bite wing x-rays

2. Angelica Green (2 hours)

   a. Periodontal Scaling (L/L & U/L)

3. Mrs. Barry (2.5 hours)

   a. PFM (tooth #29)

   b. Final Impressions for maxillary denture

4. Lynn Bacca

   a. 4-bite wing x-rays

   b. 2 anterior PAs

   c. Prophy and Fluoride Treatment

Option 2 Dentrix Independent Practice. For this exercise you will schedule the appointments listed below. Schedule all the patients for the same day. *Note:* You have already set up treatment plans for Jana Rogers, Angelica Green, and Holly Barry. Determine the provider from the list of providers that you have setup (DDS1, DDS2, HYG1, or PEDO). Decide ahead of time whether you will be assigning an operatory to specific providers. For example, does the hygienist work out of one predetermined operatory? Are there specific operatories assigned to the different providers? Refer to Scheduling (quick start) above for directions on scheduling your patients.

1. Jana Rogers (1 hour)

   a. Examination

   b. Prophy

   c. 4-bite wing x-rays

2. Angelica Green (2 hours)

   a. Periodontal Scaling (L/L & U/L)

3. Mrs. Barry (2.5 hours)

   a. PFM (tooth #29)

   b. Final Impressions for maxillary denture

4. Lynn Bacca (*Note:* You will need to check Lynn's paper chart for fees.)

   a. 4-bite wing x-rays

   b. 2 anterior PAs

   c. Prophy and Fluoride Treatment

DENTAL PRACTICE PROCEDURAL MANUAL PROJECT (OPTIONAL)

Continue working on your Dental Practice Procedural Manual (see Workbook Chapter 6 for details).
Suggested activities:

- Team meeting

- Review timeline

- Review Group research and writing assignments

- Complete research and writing assignments for this chapter

- Review and revise completed sections of the manual

- Individual journal entries

11 Continuing Care Program (Recall or Re-Care Systems)

LEARNING OBJECTIVES

1. Define recall or re-care systems.
2. Explain the benefits of a continuing care program for patients and the financial health of a dental practice, including the elements that are necessary for an effective recall system.
3. List the different classifications of recalls.
4. Identify the methods for recalling patients and explain the barriers and solutions for each method.

INTRODUCTION

A **continuing care program** is a systematic approach to encourage patients to return to the dental practice for regular examinations and prophylaxis appointments. The purpose of this approach benefits both the patient and the dental practice. The role of a dental healthcare team is to provide comprehensive, professional treatments through a system of dental examinations, preventive care measures, restorative treatments, and education. By educating patients about the benefits of home dental care and the benefits of establishing good dental health habits, the dental healthcare team forms a partnership with patients. When a team approach is used, the patient, as a team member, is more likely to accept their role in the prevention of dental disease, which includes regular examinations and prophylaxis.

EXERCISES

1. What is the function of a dental recall or re-care appointment system?

_____

_____

_____

2. List the benefits to the patient of a continuing care program.

_____

_____

_____

_____

_____

_____

_____

3. List the benefits to the dental practice of a continuing care program.

_____

_____

_____

_____

_____

_____

4. During a recall appointment, the dentist has the opportunity to reexamine the patient and evaluate his or her dental health. Identify other treatments besides prophylaxis that may require a recall appointment.

_____

_____

_____

_____

_____

_____

5. Identify the following methods of recalling patients:

a. _____ This method is highly successful because patients have personally participated in the scheduling of their own appointment.

b. _____ Requires the mailing of recall cards to patients to remind them that they are due in the dental office for an appointment.

c. _____ Requires an assistant to call each patient before the month they are due for recall to schedule the appointment.

d. _____ This method uses a data base to identify and track recall patients.

A. Automated Recall System

B. Mail Recall System

C. Prescheduled Recall System

D. Telephone Recall System

E. Tracking System

COMPUTER APPLICATION EXERCISE

What Would You Do?

Student Assignment #1

During a recent staff meeting, several issues have been raised about the effectiveness of the current recall system. The dental healthcare team has identified the following concerns:

- The hygiene schedule is booked 3 months in advance.

- There has been a decline in new patients.

- Patients are not responding to the reminder postcards that are being sent. Your task as the administrative assistant is to evaluate these concerns by identifying the problem and presenting a possible solution. You will present your findings in the form of a report at your next staff meeting.

- Type your report.

- Print a copy of the report and save to your ADA WB Chapter 11 folder.

Dentrix Learning Edition Lesson

Student Assignment #2

Go to the Evolve website and complete the Dentrix Learning Edition Lesson assignment for Chapter 11.

Lesson: Continuing Care
    Assigning Continuing Care
    Editing Continuing Care

DENTRIX APPLICATION EXERCISE (OPTIONAL)

Dentrix Learning Objectives

- Assign a continuing care plan

Dentrix User's Guide

Chapter 3: Family File

Assigning Continuing Care

Dentrix Independent Practice

1. Assign a continuing care plan for Jana Rogers, Angelica Green, Holly Barry, and Lynn Bacca.

DENTAL PRACTICE PROCEDURAL MANUAL PROJECT (OPTIONAL)

Continue working on your Dental Practice Procedural Manual (see Workbook Chapter 6 for details).
    Suggested activities:

- Team meeting

- Review timeline

- Review Group research and writing assignments

- Complete research and writing assignments for this chapter

- Review and revise completed sections of the manual

- Individual journal entries

12 Inventory Management

1. Explain how to establish a successful inventory management system, including:
   - List the information needed to order supplies and products and discuss how this information will be used.
   - Define rate of use and lead time.
   - Describe the role of an inventory manager.
   - Analyze the elements of a good inventory management system and describe how elements relate to the organization and overall effectiveness of a dental practice.
2. Identify the types of supplies, products, and equipment that are commonly purchased for a dental practice.
3. Discuss the selection and ordering process of supplies, products, and equipment, including:
   - List the information that should be considered before an order is placed for supplies and products.
   - Explain how shipments should be received and proper storage techniques.
4. Explain the role of the Occupational Safety and Health Administration (OSHA). Describe the various sections of an effective hazard communication program and discuss what information is important to an inventory manager.

INTRODUCTION

Ordering and managing supplies in a dental practice requires organization, communication, and the cooperation of the entire dental healthcare team. Inventory control is not limited to supplies in the clinical area. Those in the laboratory and business office must also be managed. Because the financial health of the dental practice depends on controlling costs, it is necessary to establish and maintain an inventory management system (IMS) that is cost effective, efficient, and easy to manage. Having the proper supplies on hand at all times is necessary in order to offer patients the best possible care.

EXERCISES

1. List the key functions of an inventory management system.

_____

_____

_____

_____

_____

_____

_____

2. List the functions and benefits of a multiservice Inventory Management Software System.

_____

_____

_____

_____

_____

_____

_____

_____

_____

3. List five characteristics of an inventory manager and write a brief statement about the one characteristic that you feel is key to the success of an IMS.

_____

_____

_____

_____

_____

4. List the different ways dental supplies and equipment can be purchased.

_____

_____

_____

_____

5. Define rate of use.

_____

_____

6. Define lead time.

_____

_____

7. Define back order.

_____

_____

8. What are your rights as a worker?

_____

_____

_____

_____

9. What are the two key administrative recommendation for an Infection Prevention Program that may be directly related to the duties of an administrative assistant or inventory manager?

_____

_____

_____

_____

_____

DENTAL PRACTICE PROCEDURAL MANUAL PROJECT (OPTIONAL)

Continue working on your Dental Practice Procedural Manual (see Workbook Chapter 6 for details).
   Suggested activities:

- Team meeting
- Review timeline
- Review Group research and writing assignments
- Complete research and writing assignments for this chapter
- Review and revise completed sections of the manual
- Individual journal entries

13 Office Equipment

LEARNING OBJECTIVES

1. List the components of a dental practice information system and explain the function of each component.
2. Describe the features and functions of a telecommunication system and explain how they can be used in a modern dental practice.
3. Compare electronic and manual systems of intraoffice communications.
4. Identify office machines commonly found in a dental practice.
5. Describe an ideal business office environment and design an ergonomic workstation.

INTRODUCTION

Business office equipment provides the tools and resources necessary to organize tasks and integrate many different functions into a seamless flow. A computer can perform many tasks using information that is maintained in a database with speed and accuracy. A telephone system integrated with a practice management software system can identify the patient and upload his or her information before the phone is answered. Cloud computing connects many devices together, from anywhere with an Internet connection. Business office equipment is selected according to the needs of the staff and the dental practice. Equipment can be divided into two broad categories: equipment used to gather, transfer, and store information; and equipment used to create a working environment that is safe, organized, and functional.

EXERCISES

1. Match the components of an information system.

Component	Function
a. Hardware ___ & ___	A. Peripheral pieces of hardware that transfer data into a computer system.
b. Input Device ___ & ___	B. Programs that allow the hardware to perform specialized tasks.
c. Output Device ___ & ___	C. People who will operate the information system
d. Software ___	D. Directions and knowledge to operate the equipment and software
e. Application software ___	E. Monitor, printer, flash drive, USB keychain driver.
f. Data ___	F. Digital imaging, bar code reader mouse, keyboard
g. Personnel ___	G. Word processing, spreadsheets, databases.
h. Procedures ___	H. Pieces of information
	I. Physical part of a computer
	J. Methods used to transfer data out of a computer
	K. CPU, mouse, keyboard, printer

2. List and briefly describe the features of a telephone system.

_____

_____

_____

_____

_____

_____

_____

3. List the functions of a telecommunication system and describe how it can be used in a dental practice.

_____

_____

_____

_____

4. List seven factors to consider when setting up an ergonomic workstation.

_____

_____

_____

_____

_____

_____

5. Match the following terms to their definitions:

a. _____ Peripheral device used to activate commands   A. CPU

b. _____ Similar to a television screen   B. Keyboard

c. _____ Information needed for the computer to be able to function   C. Mouse

d. _____ Used to back up information   D. Scanner

e. _____ Main operating component of hardware   E. Modem

f. _____ Digitizes information from a document   F. Monitor

g. _____ Produces a hard copy of information   G. Printer

h. _____ Most common input device   H. Storage device

i. _____ Transfers information   I. Operating system

6. Define intraoffice communications.

_____

7. List the different types of intraoffice communication systems.

_____

_____

_____

_____

_____

8. List the types of office machines found in a dental practice.

_____

_____

_____

_____

_____

Define the following terms:

9. Ergonomics _____

10. Background noise _____

11. Lighting _____

Ergonomic Problem Solving

12. Sally, the administrative dental assistant, is complaining of lower back pain. What should she check on her chair to rectify this problem?

_____

_____

_____

_____

13. Kevin, the business manager, is complaining of eyestrain. What can he do with his video display terminal to help alleviate the strain?

_____

_____

_____

_____

_____

14. Hope, the insurance biller, has been given a diagnosis of carpal tunnel syndrome. What can she do with her keyboard and mouse to help reduce the strain?

_____

_____

_____

_____

_____

DENTAL PRACTICE PROCEDURAL MANUAL PROJECT (OPTIONAL)

Continue working on your Dental Practice Procedural Manual (see Workbook Chapter 6 for details).
  Suggested activities:

- Team meeting
- Review timeline
- Review Group research and writing assignments
- Complete research and writing assignments for this chapter
- Review and revise completed sections of the manual
- Individual journal entries

14 Financial Arrangement and Collection Procedures

LEARNING OBJECTIVES

1. List the elements of a financial policy and discuss the qualifying factors for each of the elements.
2. Describe the different types of financial policies and explain how they can be applied in a dental practice and how they should be communicated to the patient.
3. State the purpose of managing accounts receivable, including:
   - Explain the role of the administrative dental assistant in managing accounts receivable.
   - Interpret aging reports.
   - Classify the five levels of the collection process.
   - Place a telephone collection call.
   - Process a collection letter.
   - Implement proper collection procedures.

INTRODUCTION

The responsibility for collecting fees is shared by all members of the dental healthcare team. The team will establish the policies and then follow them. The administrative dental assistant has the most visible task. After a treatment plan has been drawn up, the administrative dental assistant will write the financial plan, present the plan to the patient, and then monitor compliance with the plan. If the plan is not followed, it is usually the administrative dental assistant who initiates collection procedures.

EXERCISES

1. Match the payment plan to its definition.

a. _____ Payment is spread out over time

b. _____ Payment is paid by third-party carrier

c. _____ Payment installments are paid directly to the dental practice

d. _____ Payment is divided by length of treatment

e. _____ Another form of payment in full. Payment amount will be discounted and deposited directly into the practice's account

f. _____ Payment is made immediately after dental visit by patient

g. _____ Payment installments directed by a loan company

A. Insurance billing

B. Payment in full

C. Outside payment plan

D. In-house payment plan

E. Extended payment plan

F. Divided payment plan

G. Credit card

H. Creative payment plan

2. List the six steps to be followed in placing a telephone collection call.

_____

_____

_____

_____

_____

_____

3. At what level in the collection process should a letter be written?

   a. Level one

   b. Level two

   c. Level three

   d. Level four

   e. Level five

4. List at least two requirements of a properly written collection letter.

_____

_____

5. Match the following time intervals with the level of the collection process.

   a. _____ 0-30 days   A. Telephone reminder

   b. _____ 30-60 days   B. Ultimatum

   c. _____ 60-90 days   C. Mailed reminder

   d. _____ 90-120 days   D. Statement

   e. _____ Longer than 120 days   E. Collection letter

   f. _____ No response to letter   F. Turning of account over to collection

                                           G. Friendly reminder

COMPUTER APPLICATION EXERCISE

Student Assignment #1

Complete the Financial Arrangement form for Jana Rogers, Angelica Green, Holly Barry, and Lynn Bacca. Note: The Financial Arrangement forms were downloaded and placed in your ADA WB folder in a previous exercise or created using the paper forms at the back of the workbook. The information you will need to complete the forms is located on the Treatment Plan for each of the patients (Chapter 8) and in the following scenarios. Once the forms are completed, answer questions 1-14 below.

Jana Rogers   Angelica Green
Holly Barry   Lynn Bacca

Jana Rogers

Jana's parents both have dental insurance. After their combined benefits are calculated, it has been determined that the total benefits paid will be $1200.00.

As the administrative dental assistant, you propose the following financial arrangements.

Initial payment $75.00

Insurance estimated payment $1200.00

The balance is to be paid in three monthly payments.

Use the completed Financial Arrangement forms to answer the following questions.

1. What is the total estimate of treatment? $_____

2. What is the balance of the estimate due? $_____

3. What is the monthly payment? $_____

Angelica Green

Angelica is covered by her husband's plan. His plan will pay 60% of the total estimate of treatment. In addition, Dr. Edwards will give Angelica a 10% professional courtesy discount on the balance after the insurance estimate. It is agreed that Angelica will pay the balance in six monthly payments.

Complete a Financial Arrangement Form for Angelica, and use the information to answer the following questions.

4. What is the total estimate of treatment? $_____

5. What is the insurance estimate? $_____

6. What is the amount of the discount? $_____

7. What is the balance of the estimate due? $_____

8. What is the monthly payment? $_____

Holly Barry

Mrs. Barry is a senior citizen and will receive a 12% senior citizen discount. She has made arrangements to pay the balance in full (credit card) on April 12.

Complete a Financial Arrangement form for Mrs. Barry and use the information to answer the following questions.

9. What is the total estimate of treatment? $_____

10. What is the amount of the discount? $_____

11. What is the balance of the estimate due? $_____

Lynn Bacca

Lynn's parents both have dental insurance. The combined payment will be 100% of the total estimate for treatment, less a $50.00 deductible.

Complete a Financial Arrangement Form for Lynn and use the information to answer the following questions.

12. What is the total estimate of treatment? $_____

13. What is the insurance estimate? $_____

14. Print a copy of each of the Financial Arrangement forms and save a copy in the patient's clinical record.

Dentrix Learning Edition Lesson

Student Assignment #2

Go to the Evolve website and complete the Dentrix Learning Edition Lessons assignments for Chapter 14.
Lesson: Treatment Planning
  Getting Started with the Treatment Planner
  Creating an Alternate Case
  Updating Case Status

DENTRIX APPLICATION EXERCISE

Dentrix Student Leaning Outcomes

The student will:

- Set up a payment agreement for a family.

- Attach a note to an account.

- Print a Truth in Lending Disclosure Statement and a coupon book for scheduled payments.

User's Guide Resources

- Chapter 8: Ledger

- Setting up Financial Arrangements

- Creating Payment Agreements

- Adding Notes to the Ledger

- Creating Future Due Payment Plans

Dentrix Guided Practice

Dentrix provides you the flexibility to set up two types of financial arrangements: (1) Payment Agreements and (2) Future Due Payment Plans. Payment Agreements can be used when treatment has been completed, and the balance will be paid over time. Future Due Payment Plans can be used when treatment will be completed over time and you want to charge an account monthly.

For this exercise you will be creating a Payment Agreement for Mary Brown.

Student Assignment #3

1. In the Ledger, select a member of the family for whom you want to create a payment agreement. Select Mary Brown.

2. Click the **Billing/Payment Agreement** button or from the **File** menu, click **Billing/Payment Agreement.** The Billing/Payment Agreement Information dialogue box appears.

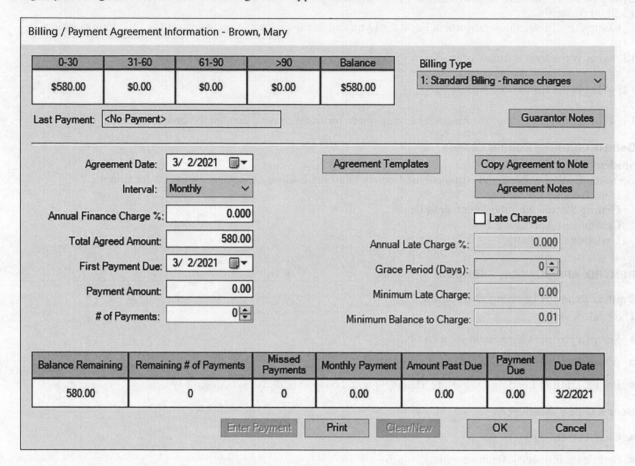

3. The current date appears in the **Agreement Date** field by default. If necessary, you can click the Down arrow to change the date of the agreement. For this exercise use today's date.

4. To apply a payment agreement template, click **Agreement Templates.** The select Payment Agreement Template dialog box appears.

Select Payment Agreement Template

Name	Finance Charge %	Late Charge %	Min Balance	Min Late Charge	Grace Period
Standard Agreement	18.000%	18.000%	$10.00	$5.00	10 days
Good Account Agreement	12.000%	12.000%	$15.00	$0.50	30 days
Collections Agreement	21.000%	21.000%	$5.00	$10.00	0 days
VIP Agreement	0.000%	0.000%	$0.01	$0.00	30 days

5. The Select Payment Agreement **Template** dialog appears, allowing you to select the payment type you want to use for the payment agreement. Select Good Account Agreement.

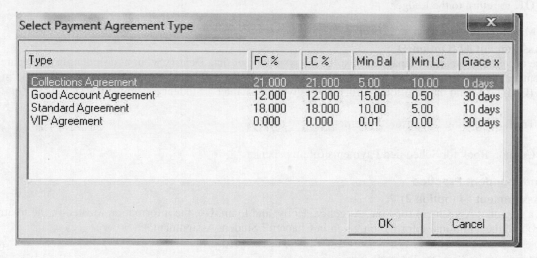

Type	FC %	LC %	Min Bal	Min LC	Grace x
Collections Agreement	21.000	21.000	5.00	10.00	0 days
Good Account Agreement	12.000	12.000	15.00	0.50	30 days
Standard Agreement	18.000	18.000	10.00	5.00	10 days
VIP Agreement	0.000	0.000	0.01	0.00	30 days

6. Click **OK** to return to the Billing/Payment Agreement Information dialog.

7. In the *Interval* group box, mark the desired interval of payments option. For this exercise check *Weekly*.

8. In the **Payment Amount** text box, type the amount of each payment. The number of payments is calculated automatically. Note: Alternately, you can set the **# of Payments** and the amount of each payment calculates automatically. For this exercise the payment will be $50 per week.

9. Enter the date that the first payment is due in the **First Pmt Due field.** For this exercise enter the date one week from today.

10. Enter the payment amount or the total number of payments in the **Payment Amt** or **Total of Payments** field. For this exercise the payment will be $25.00 per week

11. To copy the agreement information, click the **Copy Agreement to Note** button.

12. Click the **Print** button. The Print for Payment Agreement dialog box appear. Check the forms you would like to print. For this exercise check Truth in Lending Disclosure Statement and Coupon Book for Scheduled Payments (Plain Form).

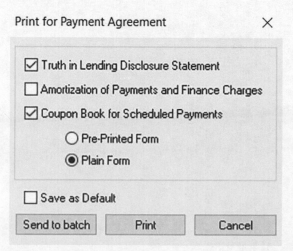

Print for Payment Agreement   ✕

☑ Truth in Lending Disclosure Statement

☐ Amortization of Payments and Finance Charges

☑ Coupon Book for Scheduled Payments

   ○ Pre-Printed Form

   ◉ Plain Form

☐ Save as Default

[Send to batch]   [Print]   [Cancel]

13. Click **Print**.

14. Click **OK** to return to the Ledger.

Practice Management Software Exercise
Student Assignment #4 (Option 1)
If you have access to a practice management software system other than Dentrix, your assignment is to prepare financial arrangement statements for your four patients, Jana, Angelica, Holly, and Lynn. Use the information located in the treatment plan (Chapter 8) and the additional information given in Chapter 7 Student Assignment #1.

A. Print a Truth in Lending Disclosure Statement.

B. Print a Coupon Book for Scheduled Payments (plain paper).

Dentrix Independent Practice
Student Assignment #4 (option 2)
Complete a Payment Agreement for Jana, Angelica, Holly, and Lynn. Use the information located in the treatment plan (Chapter 8) and the additional information given in Chapter 7 Student Assignment #1.

A. Print a Truth in Lending Disclosure Statement.

B. Print a Coupon Book for Scheduled Payments (plain paper).

DENTAL PRACTICE PROCEDURAL MANUAL PROJECT (OPTIONAL)

Continue working on your Dental Practice Procedural Manual (see Workbook Chapter 6 for details).
   Suggested activities:

- Team meeting

- Review timeline

- Review Group research and writing assignments

- Complete research and writing assignments for this chapter

- Review and revise completed sections of the manual

- Individual journal entries

15 Dental Benefit Plan Processing

LEARNING OBJECTIVES

1. Classify and identify the various types of dental benefit plans.
2. Identify the different methods of filing dental claims and discuss the responsibility of the administrative dental assistant in filing dental claims.
3. List the types of benefit plan information required to determine benefit coverage.
4. Identify the two ways that benefit plan payments can be made and discuss payment tracking.
5. Demonstrate how to complete a dental claim form.
6. Discuss the purpose of dental procedure coding and differentiate between categories.
7. Describe fraudulent benefit plan billing, including Part 5B of the American Dental Association (ADA) Code of Ethics, and identify how it applies to the administrative dental assistant.

INTRODUCTION

As the need for dental benefits has increased, so has the types of dental benefit plans and how they are funded. To help patients understand and take full advantage of their benefits, the dental healthcare team needs to understand they types of services covered, including limitations and exclusions. There are primarily two broad categories for plans: fully insured plans and self-funded plans. Within each of these plans are broad categories of plans that detail how the plan is funded, what is covered, and the fee structure.

EXERCISES

1. Match each of the following descriptions of types of dental coverage with the correct term:

   a. _____ Uses a schedule of allowance, table of allowance, or reasonable and customary fee schedule as the basis of payment calculation.

   b. _____ The employer pays for all benefits due the patient through the plan administrator.

   c. _____ The contract states that the dentist will use only the fee schedule preapproved by the third-party benefit plan.

   d. _____ Self-funded dental benefit plans that reimburse patients based on dollar spend and not the type of treatment received.

   e. _____ Publicly funded dental programs.

   f. _____ Members can receive treatment only from assigned dentists.

   g. _____ Lists of procedures covered by a benefit plan and their respective dollar amounts.

   h. _____ Fee schedules are calculated with distinct demographic information and criteria.

   i. _____ Established a marketplace, intended to lower the cost of coverage to small business and individuals.

   j. _____ Designed to contain the costs of dental procedures and services.

   k. _____ Are qualified plans that receive contributions for the purpose of providing dental benefits to participants.

   A. Fully Insured Plans

   B. Self-funded Plans

   C. Managed Care

   D. Preferred Provider Organization

   E. Health Maintenance Organization

   F. Indemnity Plans

   G. Usual, Customary, and Reasonable Plans

   H. Table of Allowances

   I. Affordable Care Act

   J. Direct Reimbursement Plans

   K. Government Programs

   L. Medicare Advantage

2. Write a short essay explaining the benefits of electronic claims processing.

_____

_____

_____

3. Dental procedure codes are:

   a. the same as medical procedure codes.

   b. set by each insurance company to correspond with its coverage.

   c. also known as SNODENT codes.

   d. standardized by the ADA and accepted by all third-party carriers.

4. Maximum coverage can be described as:

   a. the total dollar amount that will be paid for each service or procedure according to the stipulations of the insurance policy.

   b. the total dollar amount that an insurance company will pay during a year.

   c. the total dollar amount that an insurance company will pay for a family.

   d. the total dollar amount that an insurance company will pay for a lifetime.

5. The percentage of payment will vary depending on:

   a. the type of procedure.

   b. the insurance contract.

   c. where the patient seeks dental treatment.

   d. all of the above.

WHAT WOULD YOU DO?

The administrative dental assistant may be faced with many ethical and legal issues regarding the billing of insurance. In the following scenarios, use the correct reference code taken from The American Dental Association's *Principles of Ethics and Code of Professional Conduct,* Section 5B, Advisory Opinions.

6. A patient has just discovered that he will no longer be covered for insurance benefits after the end of the month. The patient is scheduled for the second week of the next month to complete his treatment plan. When you check the schedule, you discover that the dentist is taking a week off and the schedule is already overbooked. The patient asks if you can change the date to the current month so the insurance company will pay.

   a. What are your options?

   _____

   _____

   _____

   b. If you change the date, what portion of the advisory opinion addresses this issue?

   _____

7. The last staff meeting focused on ways to attract new patients to the dental practice. Several ideas were discussed. One of the ideas suggested that patients who have dental insurance would not be responsible for their copayment after the insurance company paid. Your assignment is to research the idea and report back to the group at the next meeting. What will you report back at the next meeting?

_____

_____

_____

_____

COMPUTER APPLICATION EXERCISE

For the following exercise, you will need your electronic clinical charts (or paper charts) for Jana Rogers, Angelica Green, Holly Barry, and Lynn Bacca. During the exercise you will be asked to complete an insurance claim form for each patient.

Student Assignment #1

1. Go to the Evolve website and download the assignment for Chapter 15.

2. Complete the assignment.

3. Print a copy of the completed assignment and place an electronic copy in your ADA WB Chapter 15 folder.

Dental Insurance Coding

Use the following information to complete your insurance claim forms and answer the questions.

Procedure	Dentrix Codes*
Periodic oral evaluation	X1407
Comprehensive oral evaluation	X1437
Periapical first film	X1507
Periapical each additional film	X1510
Bitewings-four	X1567
Prophylaxis-adult	X2397
Prophylaxis-child	X2490
Topical application of fluoride-child	X2495
Sealant-per tooth	X2638
Amalgam-two-surface	X3047
Crown-porcelain fused to high noble metal	X4037
Endodontic therapy, molar	X4617
Prefabricated post and core	X5237
Periodontal scaling and root planing	X5628

*The Dentrix Codes are placeholder codes designed to mimic the style of coding used by the American Dental Association (ADA). The actual ADA codes are copyrighted in the publication *Code on Dental Procedures and Nomenclature (CDT)* and appear only with the professional version of Dentrix.

Billing Dentist Information

Use the following information to complete all claim forms (all numbers are fictitious):

Mary A. Edwards, D.D.S.
4546 North Avery Way
Canyon View, CA 91783
987-555-3210
Provider ID#34567
TIN: 95-1234568
License #10111213

1. Who is responsible for primary insurance coverage for Jana Rogers?_____

2. Who is responsible for secondary insurance coverage for Jana?_____

3. Submit a completed primary insurance claim form (claim forms are located on the following pages) for Jana. Include treatment dated 12 April, 24 April, 10 May, and 17 May.

4. Who is responsible for primary insurance coverage for Angelica Green?_____

   _____

5. Identify the documentation that will be sent with Angelica's claim form._____

   _____

6. Complete a claim form for Angelica for the following dates: 6 March through 24 April. Angelica has a medical condition that may contribute to periodontal disease. ICD-10, *E08.630 Diabetes due to underlying condition with periodontal disease.*

7. Who is the responsible party for Holly Barry?_____

8. What type of insurance coverage does Holly have?_____

9. Under the birthday rule, who is responsible for primary coverage for Lynn Bacca?_____

   _____

10. When is the secondary insurance submitted for payment?_____

    _____

11. Complete a primary insurance claim form for Lynn for 12 April and 24 April.

12. Correctly document each clinical record.

ADA American Dental Association® Dental Claim Form

HEADER INFORMATION

1. Type of Transaction (Mark all applicable boxes)

☐ Statement of Actual Services   ☐ Request for Predetermination/Preauthorization

☐ EPSDT / Title XIX

2. Predetermination/Preauthorization Number

DENTAL BENEFIT PLAN INFORMATION

3. Company/Plan Name, Address, City, State, Zip Code

OTHER COVERAGE (Mark applicable box and complete items 5-11. If none, leave blank.)

4. Dental? ☐   **Medical?** ☐   (If both, complete 5-11 for dental only.)

5. Name of Policyholder/Subscriber in #4 (Last, First, Middle Initial, Suffix)

6. Date of Birth (MM/DD/CCYY)   **7. Gender** ☐M ☐F ☐U   **8. Policyholder/Subscriber ID (Assigned by Plan)**

9. Plan/Group Number   **10. Patient's Relationship to Person named in #5** ☐ Self ☐ Spouse ☐ Dependent ☐ Other

11. Other Insurance Company/Dental Benefit Plan Name, Address, City, State, Zip Code

POLICYHOLDER/SUBSCRIBER INFORMATION (Assigned by Plan Named in #3)

12. Policyholder/Subscriber Name (Last, First, Middle Initial, Suffix), Address, City, State, Zip Code

13. Date of Birth (MM/DD/CCYY)   **14. Gender** ☐M ☐F ☐U   **15. Policyholder/Subscriber ID (Assigned by Plan)**

16. Plan/Group Number   **17. Employer Name**

PATIENT INFORMATION

18. Relationship to Policyholder/Subscriber in #12 Above ☐ Self ☐ Spouse ☐ Dependent Child ☐ Other   **19. Reserved For Future Use**

20. Name (Last, First, Middle Initial, Suffix), Address, City, State, Zip Code

21. Date of Birth (MM/DD/CCYY)   **22. Gender** ☐M ☐F ☐U   **23. Patient ID/Account # (Assigned by Dentist)**

RECORD OF SERVICES PROVIDED

	24. Procedure Date (MM/DD/CCYY)	25. Area of Oral Cavity	26. Tooth System	27. Tooth Number(s) or Letter(s)	28. Tooth Surface	29. Procedure Code	29a. Diag. Pointer	29b. Qty.	30. Description	31. Fee
1										
2										
3										
4										
5										
6										
7										
8										
9										
10										

33. Missing Teeth Information (Place an "X" on each missing tooth.)

| 1 | 2 | 3 | 4 | 5 | 6 | 7 | 8 | 9 | 10 | 11 | 12 | 13 | 14 | 15 | 16 |
| 32 | 31 | 30 | 29 | 28 | 27 | 26 | 25 | 24 | 23 | 22 | 21 | 20 | 19 | 18 | 17 |

34. Diagnosis Code List Qualifier ☐ (ICD-10 = AB)

34a. Diagnosis Code(s) (Primary diagnosis in "A")

A _____   C _____

B _____   D _____

31a. Other Fee(s)

32. Total Fee

35. Remarks

AUTHORIZATIONS

36. I have been informed of the treatment plan and associated fees. I agree to be responsible for all charges for dental services and materials not paid by my dental benefit plan, unless prohibited by law, or the treating dentist or dental practice has a contractual agreement with my plan prohibiting all or a portion of such charges. To the extent permitted by law, I consent to your use and disclosure of my protected health information to carry out payment activities in connection with this claim.

X _____

Patient/Guardian Signature   Date

37. I hereby authorize and direct payment of the dental benefits otherwise payable to me, directly to the below named dentist or dental entity.

X _____

Subscriber Signature   Date

BILLING DENTIST OR DENTAL ENTITY (Leave blank if dentist or dental entity is not submitting claim on behalf of the patient or insured/subscriber.)

48. Name, Address, City, State, Zip Code

49. NPI   **50. License Number**   **51. SSN or TIN**

52. Phone Number ( ) -   **52a. Additional Provider ID**

ANCILLARY CLAIM/TREATMENT INFORMATION

38. Place of Treatment ☐ (e.g. 11=office; 22=O/P Hospital) (Use "Place of Service Codes for Professional Claims")

39. Enclosures (Y or N) ☐

40. Is Treatment for Orthodontics? ☐ No (Skip 41-42) ☐ Yes (Complete 41-42)

41. Date Appliance Placed (MM/DD/CCYY)

42. Months of Treatment

43. Replacement of Prosthesis ☐ No ☐ Yes (Complete 44)

44. Date of Prior Placement (MM/DD/CCYY)

45. Treatment Resulting from ☐ Occupational illness/injury ☐ Auto accident ☐ Other accident

46. Date of Accident (MM/DD/CCYY)   **47. Auto Accident State**

TREATING DENTIST AND TREATMENT LOCATION INFORMATION

53. I hereby certify that the procedures as indicated by date are in progress (for procedures that require multiple visits) or have been completed.

X _____

Signed (Treating Dentist)   Date

54. NPI   **55. License Number**

56. Address, City, State, Zip Code   **56a. Provider Specialty Code**

57. Phone Number ( ) -   **58. Additional Provider ID**

To reorder call 800.947.4746 or go online at ADAcatalog.org

The American Dental Association dental claim form. (Copyright © 2019 American Dental Association, Chicago, IL)

ADA American Dental Association® Dental Claim Form

HEADER INFORMATION

1. Type of Transaction (Mark all applicable boxes)

- [ ] Statement of Actual Services
- [ ] Request for Predetermination/Preauthorization
- [ ] EPSDT / Title XIX

2. Predetermination/Preauthorization Number

DENTAL BENEFIT PLAN INFORMATION

3. Company/Plan Name, Address, City, State, Zip Code

OTHER COVERAGE (Mark applicable box and complete items 5-11. If none, leave blank.)

4. Dental? [ ]   **Medical?** [ ]   (If both, complete 5-11 for dental only.)

5. Name of Policyholder/Subscriber in #4 (Last, First, Middle Initial, Suffix)

6. Date of Birth (MM/DD/CCYY)

7. Gender [ ] M [ ] F [ ] U

8. Policyholder/Subscriber ID (Assigned by Plan)

9. Plan/Group Number

10. Patient's Relationship to Person named in #5
- [ ] Self [ ] Spouse [ ] Dependent [ ] Other

11. Other Insurance Company/Dental Benefit Plan Name, Address, City, State, Zip Code

POLICYHOLDER/SUBSCRIBER INFORMATION (Assigned by Plan Named in #3)

12. Policyholder/Subscriber Name (Last, First, Middle Initial, Suffix), Address, City, State, Zip Code

13. Date of Birth (MM/DD/CCYY)

14. Gender [ ] M [ ] F [ ] U

15. Policyholder/Subscriber ID (Assigned by Plan)

16. Plan/Group Number

17. Employer Name

PATIENT INFORMATION

18. Relationship to Policyholder/Subscriber in #12 Above
- [ ] Self [ ] Spouse [ ] Dependent Child [ ] Other

19. Reserved For Future Use

20. Name (Last, First, Middle Initial, Suffix), Address, City, State, Zip Code

21. Date of Birth (MM/DD/CCYY)

22. Gender [ ] M [ ] F [ ] U

23. Patient ID/Account # (Assigned by Dentist)

RECORD OF SERVICES PROVIDED

	24. Procedure Date (MM/DD/CCYY)	25. Area of Oral Cavity	26. Tooth System	27. Tooth Number(s) or Letter(s)	28. Tooth Surface	29. Procedure Code	29a. Diag. Pointer	29b. Qty.	30. Description	31. Fee
1										
2										
3										
4										
5										
6										
7										
8										
9										
10										

33. Missing Teeth Information (Place an "X" on each missing tooth.)

1	2	3	4	5	6	7	8	9	10	11	12	13	14	15	16
32	31	30	29	28	27	26	25	24	23	22	21	20	19	18	17

34. Diagnosis Code List Qualifier [ ] (ICD-10 = AB)

34a. Diagnosis Code(s) (Primary diagnosis in "A")
A _____ C _____
B _____ D _____

31a. Other Fee(s)

32. Total Fee

35. Remarks

AUTHORIZATIONS

36. I have been informed of the treatment plan and associated fees. I agree to be responsible for all charges for dental services and materials not paid by my dental benefit plan, unless prohibited by law, or the treating dentist or dental practice has a contractual agreement with my plan prohibiting all or a portion of such charges. To the extent permitted by law, I consent to your use and disclosure of my protected health information to carry out payment activities in connection with this claim.

X _____
Patient/Guardian Signature   Date

37. I hereby authorize and direct payment of the dental benefits otherwise payable to me, directly to the below named dentist or dental entity.

X _____
Subscriber Signature   Date

BILLING DENTIST OR DENTAL ENTITY (Leave blank if dentist or dental entity is not submitting claim on behalf of the patient or insured/subscriber.)

48. Name, Address, City, State, Zip Code

49. NPI

50. License Number

51. SSN or TIN

52. Phone Number ( ) -

52a. Additional Provider ID

ANCILLARY CLAIM/TREATMENT INFORMATION

38. Place of Treatment [ ] (e.g. 11=office; 22=O/P Hospital) (Use "Place of Service Codes for Professional Claims")

39. Enclosures (Y or N) [ ]

40. Is Treatment for Orthodontics?
- [ ] No (Skip 41-42) [ ] Yes (Complete 41-42)

41. Date Appliance Placed (MM/DD/CCYY)

42. Months of Treatment

43. Replacement of Prosthesis
- [ ] No [ ] Yes (Complete 44)

44. Date of Prior Placement (MM/DD/CCYY)

45. Treatment Resulting from
- [ ] Occupational illness/injury [ ] Auto accident [ ] Other accident

46. Date of Accident (MM/DD/CCYY)

47. Auto Accident State

TREATING DENTIST AND TREATMENT LOCATION INFORMATION

53. I hereby certify that the procedures as indicated by date are in progress (for procedures that require multiple visits) or have been completed.

X _____
Signed (Treating Dentist)   Date

54. NPI

55. License Number

56. Address, City, State, Zip Code

56a. Provider Specialty Code

57. Phone Number ( ) -

58. Additional Provider ID

To reorder call 800.947.4746
or go online at ADAcatalog.org

The American Dental Association dental claim form. (Copyright © 2019 American Dental Association, Chicago, IL)

ADA American Dental Association® **Dental Claim Form**

HEADER INFORMATION

1. Type of Transaction (Mark all applicable boxes)

☐ Statement of Actual Services   ☐ Request for Predetermination/Preauthorization

☐ EPSDT / Title XIX

2. Predetermination/Preauthorization Number

DENTAL BENEFIT PLAN INFORMATION

3. Company/Plan Name, Address, City, State, Zip Code

OTHER COVERAGE (Mark applicable box and complete items 5-11. If none, leave blank.)

4. Dental? ☐   **Medical?** ☐   (If both, complete 5-11 for dental only.)

5. Name of Policyholder/Subscriber in #4 (Last, First, Middle Initial, Suffix)

6. Date of Birth (MM/DD/CCYY)   **7. Gender** ☐ M ☐ F ☐ U   **8. Policyholder/Subscriber ID** (Assigned by Plan)

9. Plan/Group Number   **10. Patient's Relationship to Person named in #5** ☐ Self ☐ Spouse ☐ Dependent ☐ Other

11. Other Insurance Company/Dental Benefit Plan Name, Address, City, State, Zip Code

POLICYHOLDER/SUBSCRIBER INFORMATION (Assigned by Plan Named in #3)

12. Policyholder/Subscriber Name (Last, First, Middle Initial, Suffix), Address, City, State, Zip Code

13. Date of Birth (MM/DD/CCYY)   **14. Gender** ☐ M ☐ F ☐ U   **15. Policyholder/Subscriber ID** (Assigned by Plan)

16. Plan/Group Number   **17. Employer Name**

PATIENT INFORMATION

18. Relationship to Policyholder/Subscriber in #12 Above ☐ Self ☐ Spouse ☐ Dependent Child ☐ Other   **19. Reserved For Future Use**

20. Name (Last, First, Middle Initial, Suffix), Address, City, State, Zip Code

21. Date of Birth (MM/DD/CCYY)   **22. Gender** ☐ M ☐ F ☐ U   **23. Patient ID/Account #** (Assigned by Dentist)

RECORD OF SERVICES PROVIDED

	24. Procedure Date (MM/DD/CCYY)	25. Area of Oral Cavity	26. Tooth System	27. Tooth Number(s) or Letter(s)	28. Tooth Surface	29. Procedure Code	29a. Diag. Pointer	29b. Qty.	30. Description	31. Fee
1										
2										
3										
4										
5										
6										
7										
8										
9										
10										

33. Missing Teeth Information (Place an "X" on each missing tooth.)

1 2 3 4 5 6 7 8 9 10 11 12 13 14 15 16

32 31 30 29 28 27 26 25 24 23 22 21 20 19 18 17

34. Diagnosis Code List Qualifier ☐ (ICD-10 = AB)

34a. Diagnosis Code(s) (Primary diagnosis in "A")   A _____   C _____   B _____   D _____

31a. Other Fee(s)

32. Total Fee

35. Remarks

AUTHORIZATIONS

36. I have been informed of the treatment plan and associated fees. I agree to be responsible for all charges for dental services and materials not paid by my dental benefit plan, unless prohibited by law, or the treating dentist or dental practice has a contractual agreement with my plan prohibiting all or a portion of such charges. To the extent permitted by law, I consent to your use and disclosure of my protected health information to carry out payment activities in connection with this claim.

X _____
Patient/Guardian Signature   Date

37. I hereby authorize and direct payment of the dental benefits otherwise payable to me, directly to the below named dentist or dental entity.

X _____
Subscriber Signature   Date

BILLING DENTIST OR DENTAL ENTITY (Leave blank if dentist or dental entity is not submitting claim on behalf of the patient or insured/subscriber.)

48. Name, Address, City, State, Zip Code

49. NPI   **50. License Number**   **51. SSN or TIN**

52. Phone Number ( ) -   **52a. Additional Provider ID**

ANCILLARY CLAIM/TREATMENT INFORMATION

38. Place of Treatment ☐ (e.g. 11=office; 22=O/P Hospital) (Use "Place of Service Codes for Professional Claims")   **39. Enclosures (Y or N)** ☐

40. Is Treatment for Orthodontics? ☐ No (Skip 41-42) ☐ Yes (Complete 41-42)   **41. Date Appliance Placed (MM/DD/CCYY)**

42. Months of Treatment   **43. Replacement of Prosthesis** ☐ No ☐ Yes (Complete 44)   **44. Date of Prior Placement (MM/DD/CCYY)**

45. Treatment Resulting from ☐ Occupational illness/injury ☐ Auto accident ☐ Other accident

46. Date of Accident (MM/DD/CCYY)   **47. Auto Accident State**

TREATING DENTIST AND TREATMENT LOCATION INFORMATION

53. I hereby certify that the procedures as indicated by date are in progress (for procedures that require multiple visits) or have been completed.

X _____
Signed (Treating Dentist)   Date

54. NPI   **55. License Number**

56. Address, City, State, Zip Code   **56a. Provider Specialty Code**

57. Phone Number ( ) -   **58. Additional Provider ID**

The American Dental Association dental claim form. (Copyright © 2019 American Dental Association, Chicago, IL)

Dentrix Learning Edition Lessons
Student Assignment #2

Go to the Evolve website and complete the Dentrix Learning Edition Lessons for Chapter 15.
Lesson: Insurance:
    Assigning Primary Insurance to a Patient
    Assigning Secondary Insurance to a Patient
    Creating a Primary Insurance Claim
    Creating a Secondary Insurance Claim

DENTRIX APPLICATION EXERCISE

Dentrix Student Learning Outcomes

The student will:

- Create an insurance claim.

- Add attachments or add other required information into an insurance claim.

- Place notations on an insurance claim.

- Print an insurance claim.

Dentrix User's Guide Resources

Chapter 8: Ledger

    Processing Insurance Claims

    Creating Primary Dental Insurance Claims

    Changing Claim Information

    Printing insurance claims

Dentrix Guided Practice

Processing insurance claims is a major component of Dentrix. Dentrix provides many tools and features that help organize and simplify the insurance claims process. From the *Family File* you are able to enter new insurance plans and assign insurance to subscriber and non-subscribers when creating or editing patient records (these procedures were explained in Chapter 8). From the *Ledger* you will be able to create primary dental insurance claims, change claim information, and edit or delete claims. You will also be able to post insurance payments and submit claims for payment from secondary insurance. From the *Office Manager* you will be able to batch process the submission of dental claims. With multilabel ways to gather and review information you will be able to communicate information to the patient about their benefits used and deductibles met.

Creating Insurance Claims

When work has been completed and is posted in the Ledger, you can create a primary insurance claim for the procedures.

Student Assignment #3

1. In the Ledger select a patient. For this exercise select Mary Brown.

2. Create the insurance claim.

If the procedures for the claim were posted on another day, select the procedures that you want to create a claim for, and then, from the **Insurance** menu, click **Selected Procedures**. For this exercise you will select all of the procedures for Mary.

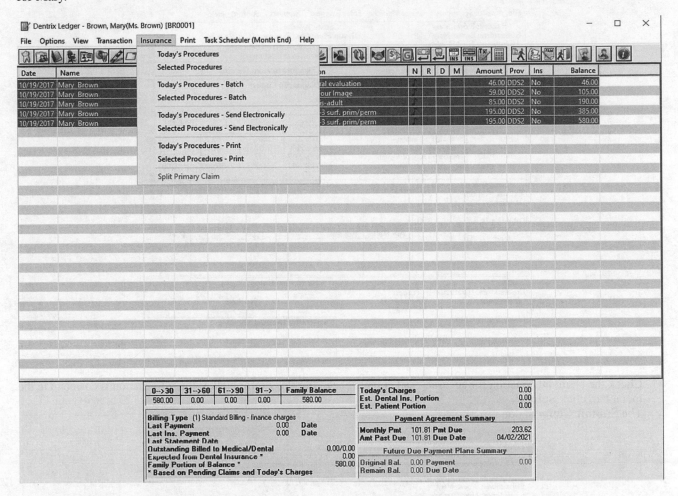

If the procedures for the claim were posted today, from the **Insurance** menu click **Today's Procedures**.
(You will use this method for the exercises in Chapter 17)

Tip: When you have multiple procedures to include, hold the right mouse button or press the Ctrl key and click each procedure to be included on the claim with the left mouse button.

The Primary Dental Insurance Claim Window appears.

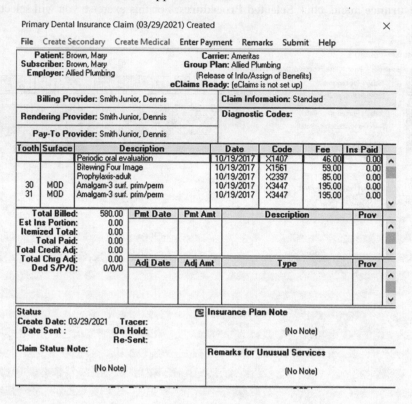

3. Check the claim information for accuracy and completeness. For this exercise all of the information is correct. On the menu bar, click **Submit**.
The **Submit Claim** dialog box appears.

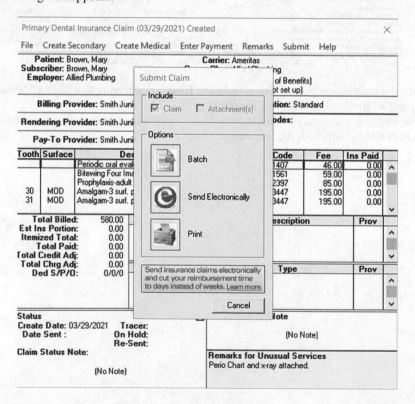

4. Click the **Print** button to print a copy of Mary's insurance claim.

Important: You must select one of the three buttons before exiting the Primary Dental Insurance Claim window to prevent the claim from staying on the account without getting submitted.

Adding additional information to a claim

When insurance claims require additional information such as student status, attachments, reason for preauthorization, additional insurance information, or other information, you will need to add the information to the claim. You can add or edit information from the Primary Dental Insurance Claim window, which you can open from the Ledger. To open the window, you can double click an existing claim, or the window will open when you process a dental insurance claim.

Student Assignment #4

1. In the Ledger, select a patient. For this exercise select Carol Little.

2. Select the procedure (endo therapy) and create an insurance claim. The Primary Dental Insurance Claim window appears.

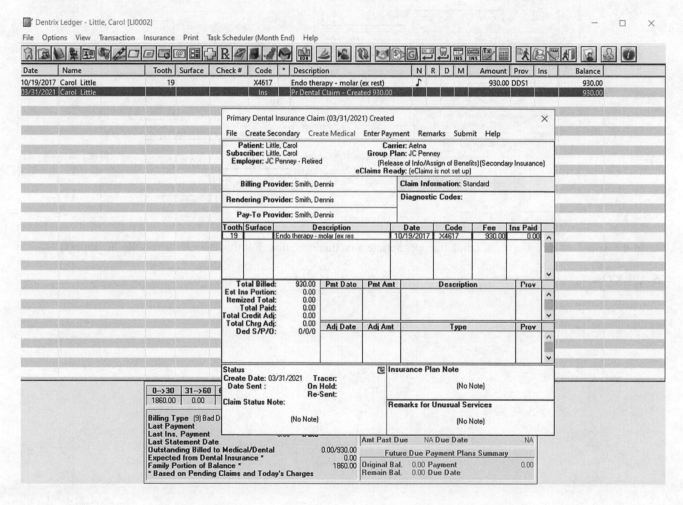

3. From the Primary Dental Insurance window double click the **Claim Information** block. The Insurance Claim Information dialog box appears.

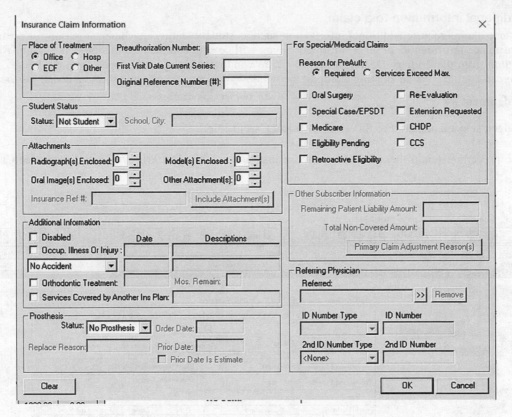

4. In the *Attachments* group box, chick the appropriate attachment option. For this exercise check Radiograph(s) 1.

5. Click **OK**.

6. From the Primary Dental Insurance Claim window click **Remarks** and the **Remarks for Unusual Services** window opens, click **Claim Remarks** select **X-ray attachment**.

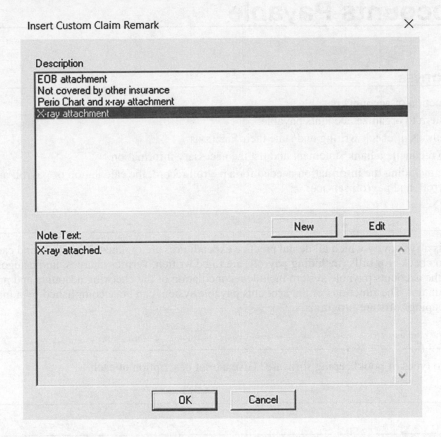

7. Click **OK**.

8. Click **OK** to close the Remarks for Unusual Services window and return to the Primary Dental Insurance window.

9. Click **Submit** and print a copy of the claim. The notation will appear on the printed claim.

Practice Management Software Exercise

Student Assignment #4 (option 1). If you have access to a practice management software system other than Dentrix, your assignment is to review the insurance information for your patients Jana, Angelica, and Lynn. Using the information from Chapter 8 verify that all the insurance information for primary and secondary insurance has been entered. Correct or edit as needed. You will be using this information to complete assignments in Chapter 17.

Dentrix Independent Practice

Student Assignment #4 (option 2). For this exercise you will review the family records you have created in Dentrix (Rogers, Green, and Bacca). Using the information you were given in Chapter 8 verify that all of the insurance information for primary and secondary insurance has been entered. Correct or edit as needed (from the *Family File*). You will be using this information to complete assignments in Chapter 17.

Tip: You may find it helpful to review the Dentrix Users Guide, Chapter 3 **Family File** (Insurance).

131

16 Bookkeeping Procedures: Accounts Payable

LEARNING OBJECTIVES

1. Describe the function of accounts payable.
2. Formulate a system to organize accounts payable.
3. Analyze the methods of check writing and state their functions.
4. Discuss steps to reconcile a bank statement and list the necessary information.
5. Discuss payroll, including the information needed for a payroll record, the calculation of payroll and necessary taxes, reporting of payroll, and payroll services.

INTRODUCTION

Accounts payable is a system by which all dental practice expenditures are organized, verified, and categorized. The system identifies when checks for bills (including payroll) are to be written, verifies charges, and categorizes expenditures. Other elements of the accounts payable system include reconciliation of the checking accounts and preparation of documents for the accountant. The functions of the accounts payable system can be accomplished by a manual bookkeeping or by using bookkeeping software programs.

EXERCISES

1. What are the two types of bookkeeping software? Give a brief description of each.

   a. _____

   b. _____

2. Why is it important to have an accounts payable system?

   _____

   _____

   _____

   _____

   _____

3. What does EFT stand for? Give three examples.

   _____

   _____

4. What is the difference between an invoice and a statement?

_____

_____

_____

_____

_____

5. List the steps required to reconcile a checking account.

_____

_____

_____

_____

_____

6. When a checking account does no balance, what are you looking for when you double check all addition and subtraction entries?

_____

_____

_____

_____

_____

7. What is needed to create a payroll record for a new employee?

   a. _____

   b. _____

   c. _____

ACTIVITY EXERCISE

For the following exercises, you will be calculating payroll and writing a check.

   Scenario: Your payroll system is offline today, and you need to calculate payroll for Sue Smith. During the process you will calculate the total hours worked, calculate payroll deductions, fill in the information on her payroll record, and write a check.

1. Total the hours worked for Sue Smith: What are the total hours worked? _____

Time Card

Employee: Sue Smith

Pay period: 4/1 to 4/13

Date	Time in	Time out	Time in	Time out	Total Hours
4/1	8:00	12:00	1:30	5:30	
4/2	8:00	12:00	1:00	5:00	
4/3	10:00	1:00	2:00	6:00	
4/5	7:45	12:15	1:30	5:00	
4/6	7:30	1:30			
4/9	8:00	12:00	1:30	5:30	
4/10	8:00	12:00	1:00	5:00	
4/11	10:00	1:00	2:00	6:00	
4/12	7:45	12:15	1:30	5:00	
4/13	7:30	1:30			
TOTAL HOURS WORKED					

Marital status **M**
Number of Exp **1**

EMPLOYEE'S PAYROLL RECORD

Name: **Sue Smith**   Social Security Number: **620-31-8752**
Address: **18 N. Fox Glenn**   City: **CanyonView**   Zip code: _____
Telephone: **555-3816**   Date of birth: **06/20/70**
Occupation: **Dental Assistant**   Date of employment: **10/2**
Pay rate: **$26.50**

Date	Check number	Gross salary	Fed W/H	FICA	M/C	State W/H	Other	Net check
Total								

2. Refer to Sue's payroll record above for the following information:

Marital Status   a. _____
Exemptions   b. _____
Rate of Pay   c. _____

3. Calculate the following for Sue Smith:

Gross Salary (Refer to Sue's payroll record and the time card to calculate.)
total hours worked x rate of pay   a. $ _____
Federal Withholding (See Tax Table)   b. $ _____
FICA Tax (6.2%)   c. $ _____
Medicare (1.45%)   d. $ _____
401k (6%)   e. $ _____

4. Complete the payroll record (using your calculations in question #3) and calculate the net salary (take home) for Sue.
   a. Net Salary $_____

   Gross salary – Fed w/h – FICA – M/C – State w/h (none) – other (401k) = net salary

Wage Bracket Method Tables for Income Tax Withholding

MARRIED Persons—SEMIMONTHLY Payroll Period

(For Wages Paid through December 2019)

And the wages are—		And the number of withholding allowances claimed is—										
At least	But less than	0	1	2	3	4	5	6	7	8	9	10
		The amount of income tax to be withheld is—										
1,362	1,382	89	71	53	36	18	1	0	0	0	0	0
1,382	1,402	92	73	55	38	20	3	0	0	0	0	0
1,402	1,422	94	75	57	40	22	5	0	0	0	0	0
1,422	1,442	97	77	59	42	24	7	0	0	0	0	0
1,442	1,462	99	79	61	44	26	9	0	0	0	0	0
1,462	1,482	101	81	63	46	28	11	0	0	0	0	0
1,482	1,502	104	83	65	48	30	13	0	0	0	0	0
1,502	1,522	106	85	67	50	32	15	0	0	0	0	0
1,522	1,542	109	88	69	52	34	17	0	0	0	0	0
1,542	1,562	111	90	71	54	36	19	1	0	0	0	0
1,562	1,582	113	92	73	56	38	21	3	0	0	0	0
1,582	1,602	116	95	75	58	40	23	5	0	0	0	0
1,602	1,622	118	97	77	60	42	25	7	0	0	0	0
1,622	1,642	121	100	79	62	44	27	9	0	0	0	0
1,642	1,662	123	102	81	64	46	29	11	0	0	0	0
1,662	1,682	125	104	83	66	48	31	13	0	0	0	0
1,682	1,702	128	107	86	68	50	33	15	0	0	0	0
1,702	1,722	130	109	88	70	52	35	17	0	0	0	0
1,722	1,742	133	112	91	72	54	37	19	2	0	0	0
1,742	1,762	135	114	93	74	56	39	21	4	0	0	0
1,762	1,782	137	116	95	76	58	41	23	6	0	0	0
1,782	1,802	140	119	98	78	60	43	25	8	0	0	0
1,802	1,822	142	121	100	80	62	45	27	10	0	0	0
1,822	1,842	145	124	103	82	64	47	29	12	0	0	0
1,842	1,862	147	126	105	84	66	49	31	14	0	0	0
1,862	1,882	149	128	107	86	68	51	33	16	0	0	0
1,882	1,902	152	131	110	89	70	53	35	18	0	0	0
1,902	1,922	154	133	112	91	72	55	37	20	2	0	0
1,922	1,942	157	136	115	94	74	57	39	22	4	0	0
1,942	1,962	159	138	117	96	76	59	41	24	6	0	0
1,962	1,982	161	140	119	98	78	61	43	26	8	0	0
1,982	2,002	164	143	122	101	80	63	45	28	10	0	0
2,002	2,022	166	145	124	103	82	65	47	30	12	0	0
2,022	2,042	169	148	127	106	85	67	49	32	14	0	0
2,042	2,062	171	150	129	108	87	69	51	34	16	0	0
2,062	2,082	173	152	131	110	89	71	53	36	18	1	0
2,082	2,102	176	155	134	113	92	73	55	38	20	3	0
2,102	2,122	178	157	136	115	94	75	57	40	22	5	0
2,122	2,142	181	160	139	118	97	77	59	42	24	7	0
2,142	2,162	183	162	141	120	99	79	61	44	26	9	0
2,162	2,182	185	164	143	122	101	81	63	46	28	11	0
2,182	2,202	188	167	146	125	104	83	65	48	30	13	0
2,202	2,222	190	169	148	127	106	85	67	50	32	15	0
2,222	2,242	193	172	151	130	109	88	69	52	34	17	0
2,242	2,262	195	174	153	132	111	90	71	54	36	19	1
2,262	2,282	197	176	155	134	113	92	73	56	38	21	3
2,282	2,302	200	179	158	137	116	95	75	58	40	23	5
2,302	2,322	202	181	160	139	118	97	77	60	42	25	7
2,322	2,342	205	184	163	142	121	100	79	62	44	27	9
2,342	2,362	207	186	165	144	123	102	81	64	46	29	11
2,362	2,382	209	188	167	146	125	104	83	66	48	31	13
2,382	2,402	212	191	170	149	128	107	86	68	50	33	15
2,402	2,422	214	193	172	151	130	109	88	70	52	35	17
2,422	2,442	217	196	175	154	133	112	91	72	54	37	19
2,442	2,462	219	198	177	156	135	114	93	74	56	39	21
2,462	2,482	221	200	179	158	137	116	95	76	58	41	23
2,482	2,502	224	203	182	161	140	119	98	78	60	43	25
2,502	2,522	226	205	184	163	142	121	100	80	62	45	27
2,522	2,542	229	208	187	166	145	124	103	82	64	47	29
2,542	2,562	231	210	189	168	147	126	105	84	66	49	31
2,562	2,582	233	212	191	170	149	128	107	86	68	51	33
2,582	2,602	236	215	194	173	152	131	110	89	70	53	35
2,602	2,622	238	217	196	175	154	133	112	91	72	55	37
2,622	2,642	241	220	199	178	157	136	115	94	74	57	39
2,642	2,662	243	222	201	180	159	138	117	96	76	59	41
2,662	2,682	245	224	203	182	161	140	119	98	78	61	43

2,682 and over   Use Table 3(b) for a MARRIED person on page 46. Also see the instructions on page 44.

5. Write a payroll check for Sue Smith.

Mary A. Edwards, D.D.S.
4546 North Avery Way
Canyon View, CA 91783

YOUR BANK HERE
CITY, STATE ZIP

00-0000
0000

No. 3223

PAY _____ DOLLARS

TO THE
ORDER OF _____

DISC.	DATE	CHECK NO.	AMOUNT	
			DOLLARS	CTS.

YOUR NAME HERE

⑈OO⅃854⑈ ⑇OOOOOOOOO⑇ OOOOOOO⑈

17 Bookkeeping Procedures: Accounts Receivable

LEARNING OBJECTIVES

1. Explain the role of the administrative dental assistant in the management of patient financial transactions.
2. Identify the components of financial records organization.
3. Perform the steps in the daily routine for managing patient transactions.
4. List and explain the types of financial reports used in a dental office.

INTRODUCTION

Dentistry, like any business, is mandated by federal and state regulations to maintain a system that documents the collection of monies. Smart business practice also requires that a financial system be maintained, with both accounts receivable and accounts payable. Accounts receivable is the system that records all financial transactions between a patient and the dental practice. This system calculates the amount of money owed to the dental practice by accounting for charges and payments. Accounts payable is the system that records all monies the dental practice owes others. It is the responsibility of the administrative dental assistant to maintain accurate records in the management of accounts receivable and accounts payable.

EXERCISES

1. Describe the routine for managing financial transactions.

_____

_____

_____

_____

_____

_____

_____

2. Explain the purpose of an audit report.

_____

_____

3. List the types of reports and identify their primary use in a dental practice.

_____

_____

_____

_____

_____

_____

_____

COMPUTER APPLICATION EXERCISE

Dentrix Learning Edition Lessons
Student Assignment #1
Go to the Evolve website and complete the Dentrix Learning Edition Lessons assignments for Chapter 17.
Lesson: Billing and Accounts Receivable
    Getting Started with the Ledger
    Posting and Editing a Procedure in the Ledger
Lesson: Insurance
    Posting Insurance Payment
Lesson: Scheduling
    Setting an Appointment Complete
Lesson: Reporting
    Getting Started with the Office Manager
    Generating a Day Sheet
    Generating an Aging Report

DENTRIX APPLICATION EXERCISE

Dentrix Student Learning Outcomes
The student will:

- Complete appointments.

- Post transactions.

- Perform task for patients from the time they check-in until the check-out.

- Perform daily practice management routines.

- Perform end of day tasks.

- As part of the daily routine you will perform a series of tasks that will organize the day, track patient treatment, post patient transactions, check out a patient, and schedule new appointments.

Dentrix User's Guide Resources

Dentrix Guided Practice

Student Assignment #2

Before you can complete the following tasks, it will be necessary to move the patients you scheduled during the Dentrix Appointment Book Chapter 10 exercise to the current day in the appointment book (instructions to follow). If you have not scheduled patients, you can select patients from the Appointment List in the Appointment Book module (Appt List> Select List drop-down, Unscheduled).

Moving Appointments

Whether a patient needs to reschedule or the office needs to lighten the schedule, from time to time you will need to move an already scheduled appointment to a new date or time. You can either move an appointment directly to a new date and time or move it temporarily to the Pinboard. *Note:* You can move appointments in Day View and Week View but not in Month View.

Moving an appointment directly to a new date and time

1. In the Appointment Book module, set the Day View or Week View, depending on whether you are moving the appointment to a different time in the same day or to a different day of the same week.

2. In Appointment Book, click the appointment that you want to move and drag it to the new date.

3. When the **Move Appointment** message appears, click **Yes.**

Moving an appointment to the Pinboard

1. In the Appointment Book, click the appointment that you want to move and drag it to the Pinboard of the Appointment Book.

2. Find a new date and time for the appointment.

3. Click the appointment icon on the Pinboard and drag the appointment to the new date and time.

4. When the **Move Appointment** message appears, click **Yes.**

    Tip: If you know the exact date and time to which you want to move an appointment, double click the appointment to open the **Appointment Information** dialogue box, enter the new date and time in the date and time fields, and click **OK.**

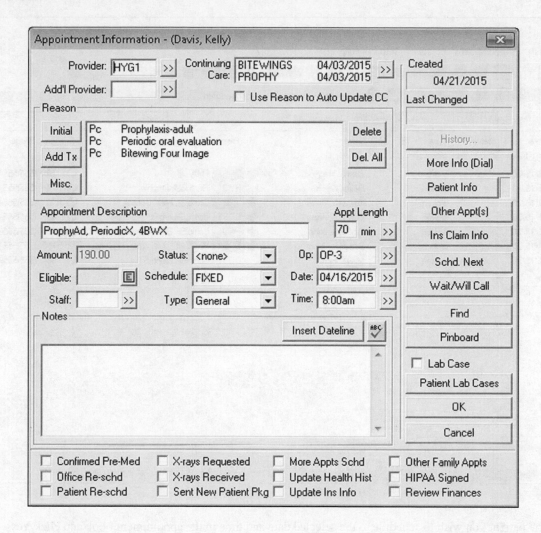

Moving an appointment from a list

1. In the Appointment Book, click Appt List and select the list you wish to use. For this exercise use the Unscheduled List.

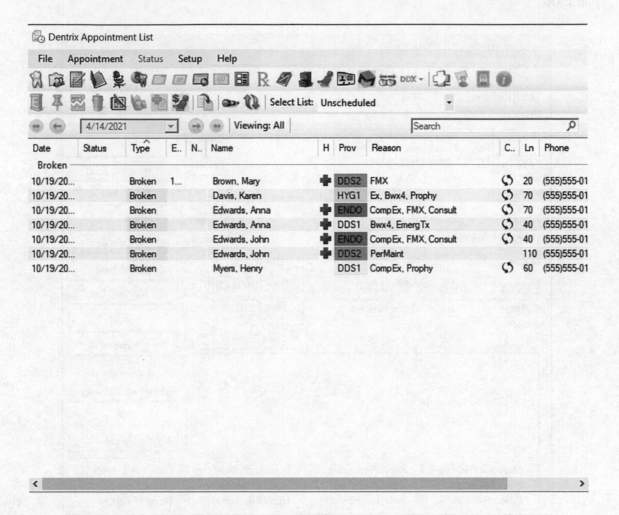

2. Drag the patient you wish to schedule to the selected date and time in the appointment book and click **Yes**.

Route Slips

The Dentrix Route Slip can be used for a variety of information purposes: as a reminder of Medical Alerts, for patient notes, and for collection information for patients being seen that day. Also, all future appointments for every family member appear on the Patient Route Slip. To generate a route slip:

1. From the Appointment Book, select an appointment (single click).

2. From the Appointment Book toolbar, click the **Print Route Slip** button (or left click to open a menu of options). The Print Route Slip dialogue box appears.

3. To print the report immediately, click the **Print** button.

Checking in a Patient When a patient arrives in the dental office, you will be able to change the status of the patient and alert team members that their patient has arrived and is ready to be seen. You will also need to check the patient's file for any alerts and changes in information and medical history. All of these tasks can be completed directly from the Appointment Information dialogue box.

1. Double click the selected patient in the appointment book. The Appointment Information dialogue box will appear (see previous Appointment Information box).

   ■ In the Appointment Description group box you can change the status. From the **Status** drop-down select **Here**

   Note: The selections in the Status box drop-down include a wide range of messages such as: patient confirmed (FIRM), if it is an emergency appointment (EMER), if the patient has arrived (HERE). This is a method used to let you or any viewer know where you are in the appointment process and is an excellent communication tool.

2. Click OK when you are finished.

Posting Scheduled Work

Once an appointment has been completed, you can quickly post procedures attached to the appointment with the click of one button. To post appointment procedures:

1. In the Appointment Book, select the Appointment you want to post as complete.

2. From the Appointment Book toolbar (or left click and select **Post/Set Complete**), click the **Set Complete** button. The Set Appointment Procedures Complete dialogue box appears.

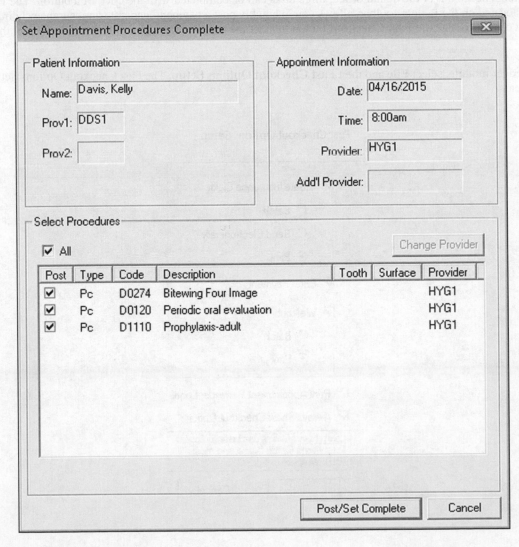

3. All procedures attached to the appointment are highlighted. If a procedure has not been completed on this visit, click it once to remove the checked box. *Note:* If the patient has had additional treatment completed during the visit, post the work in the Chart or Ledger.

4. Click the **Post/Set Complete** button in the Set Appointment Complete dialog box. The procedures are posted to the Chart/Ledger, and the appointment turns gray, indicating that it has been completed.

Scheduling the Next Appointment

1. Left-click on the patient in the Appointment Book.

2. Click Other Appointments.

3. Select the treatment to be scheduled.

4. Click Create New Appt.

5. Complete the **Appointment Information** dialogue box. (*Reason* group box and *Appointment Description* group box, Date and Time.

6. Click **OK** (this will take you to the day and time you selected, if this is correct return to the current date.)

Fast Checkout Button

When a patient checks out of the dental office, three tasks can be completed with the click of a button. The **Fast Checkout** button, located on the Ledger toolbar, allows you to quickly post a payment, generate an insurance claim, and print a receipt. You can customize the **Fast Checkout** button to meet the needs of the office. For this exercise, set the following options:

1. In the Ledger module, select **File** and then **Fast Checkout Options Setup.** The Fast Checkout Options Setup dialogue box appears.

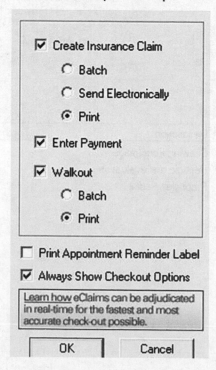

Fast Checkout Options Setup

2. Set up the following tasks:

   a. Click Create Insurance Claim; then select Print.

   b. Click Enter Payment.

   c. Click **Walkout,** and then select **Print.**

   d. Click Always Show Checkout options.

   e. Click **OK.**

Using fast checkout

1. From the appointment book Left click the selected patient. Click **Ledger**.

2. If you have not already posted the procedures for this patient, post them at this time.

3. From the Ledger toolbar, click the **Fast Checkout** button. If you have set the button option to always show Checkout Options, the Checkout Options Setup dialogue box appears.

4. Select the desired option(s) if necessary.

5. Click **OK.**

6. The Enter Payment dialogue box appears. Enter the payment information and click **OK.**

Enter Payment

Date:	4/14/2021
Amount:	0.00
Check/Payment #:	
Bank/Branch #:	
Provider:	Split By Provider
Patient:	Brown, Mary * (Ms. Brown) [Bf
Split Method:	Guarantor Estimate

Search

Payment Types
- Check Payment - Thank You
- Cash Payment - Thank You
- VISA Payment - Thank You
- MasterCard Payment -Thank You
- Discover Payment - Thank You
- AMEX Payment - Thank You
- Pre-Dentrix Ins Pmt- Thank You

☑ Apply To Payment Agreement

▶ Details

▶ Note

Settings ⚙

⚠   OK   Cancel

End-of-Day Tasks

At the end of each day you will need to complete all posting of daily transactions, prepare a bank deposit, generate a Day Sheet Report, complete insurance processing, and account for all transactions.

Generate a day sheet report

The Day Sheet shows all transactions entered in your database for a given date range. To generate a Day sheet:

1. In the Office Manager, select **Reports>Management>Day Sheets (Charges and Receipts)** or click the Day Sheet Report button. The Day Sheet dialog box appears.

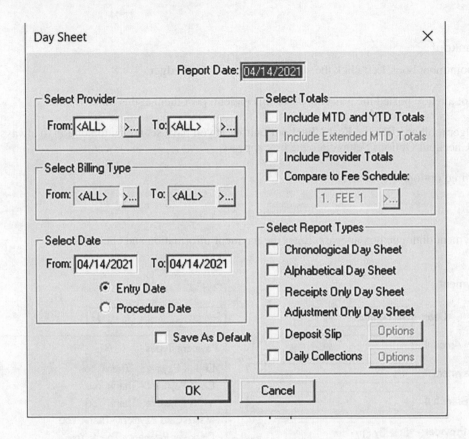

2. In the *Select Provider* group box, select the desired provider range. For this exercise select all.

3. In the *Select Billing Type* group box, select the desired billing type range. For this exercise select all.

4. In the *Select Date* group box, enter the desired date range and mark the desired options. The default is set with today's date, change the date if different. *Note:* You have to have procedures posted before you can generate a day sheet.

5. In the *Select Totals* group box, check the desired options: For this exercise select MTD and YTD totals and include provider totals.

6. In the *Select Report Type* group box, check the desired options: For this exercise select *Chronological, Deposit Slip* (option select ALL), *Daily Collections* (options select ALL).

7. Click **OK** to send the report to the Batch Processor and return to the Office Manager.

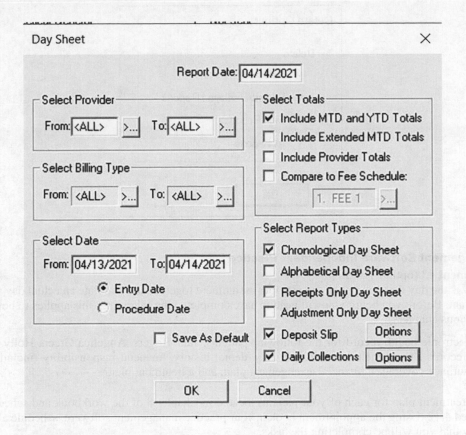

Preview reports in the Batch Processor
To preview reports you have sent to the Batch Processor.

1. Select the report in the Batch Processor.

2. Click the Preview Button.

Print reports in the Batch Processor
To print reports you have sent to the Batch Processor.

1. Select the report in the Batch Processor.

2. Click the **Print Report(s)** button.

Delete reports from the Batch Processor
When reports are no longer needed, it will be necessary to clear them from the Batch Processor.

1. Select the report in the Batch Processor.

2. Click the **Delete Report(s)** button. The Delete Options dialog appears.

3. In the *Delete* group box, mark the desired option.

4. Click **OK**.

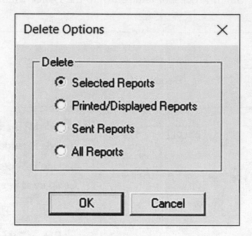

Practice Management Software Independent Practice

Student Assignment #3 (option 1 and 2)

Scenario: Today is the day that you put all the previous assignment together and simulate an actual day as an administrative dental assistant. Before you begin you will need to have completed the following (this applies to both option 1 and 2 exercises in previous chapters).

1. Created an electronic health record for the following patients: Jana Rogers, Angelica Green, Holly Barry, and Lynn Bacca. Your records should include medical history, dental history, financial responsibility (including primary and secondary insurance coverage), financial arrangement plan, and a treatment plan.

2. Refer to the treatment plan for each of your patients located in Chapter 8 of the workbook and schedule them for the treatment dated 4/12. Using the appointment book in your practice management software, schedule all the patients for the actual day that you will be completing the tasks.

As your day progresses, you will have:

1. Printed a copy of the appointment book view to place in each treatment rooms.

2. Created routing slips for each of your patients.

3. Checked in your patient as they arrive for their appointment.

4. Posted completed treatment.

5. Scheduled their next appointment (refer to their treatment plan for addition work dated after 4/12).

6. Collected the following payments.

   a. Jana Rogers - $75 check

   b. Angelica Green - $125.00 check

   c. Holly Barry – credit card payment per her financial agreement

   d. Lynn Bacca - $50.00 cash

7. Printed an insurance claim for each patient.

8. Printed a walkout statement (statement of services rendered) for each patient.

9. Printed end of day reports.

    a. Day sheet report

    b. Deposit slip report

    c. Insurance report

    d. Daily collections report

18 Employment Strategies

LEARNING OBJECTIVES

1. List career opportunities for administrative dental assistants.
2. Identify and explain the steps to be followed in developing an employment strategy. Discuss the function of each step, including:
   - Construct a high-quality resume and cover letter.
   - Identify the avenues of where to look for employment.
   - Explain the function of a personal career portfolio and discuss its advantages.
   - Identify and respond to common interview questions.
   - Explain the proper way to accept and leave a job.

INTRODUCTION

Hundreds of jobs are waiting for the right person to fill them. The hiring decision is based on the ability of the prospective employee to successfully present himself or herself. Convincing the employer that you are the best person for the job is not easy. The process begins with a self-study and ends with a personal interview. Along the way, you will identify career options, answer questions about yourself, research possible employment opportunities, produce a quality resume, construct a letter of introduction, complete an application, and prepare mentally and physically for an interview.

EXERCISES

1. List the career opportunities for an administrative dental assistant.

_____

_____

_____

_____

_____

2. List and state the purpose of the steps involved in developing employment strategies.

_____

_____

_____

_____

_____

_____

3. What will a strong resume tell the reader about you?

_____

_____

_____

_____

4. List the components of a quality resume.

_____

_____

_____

_____

_____

_____

5. Describe the function of a personal career portfolio.

_____

_____

_____

_____

_____

6. List the components of a personal career portfolio.

_____

_____

_____

_____

_____

_____

7. List the components of a quality resume.

_____

_____

_____

_____

_____

_____

8. List the various avenues that may lead to employment.

_____

_____

_____

_____

_____

_____

COMPUTER APPLICATION EXERCISE

Student Assignment #1

1. Select a resume style (a chronological resume, a functional resume, or a hybrid resume) and produce a high-quality resume.

2. Write a cover letter.

Student Assignment #2

Go to the Evolve website and download the assignment for Chapter 18.

1. Complete the assignment.

2. Print a copy of the completed assignment and place an electronic copy in your ADA WB Chapter 18 folder.

DENTAL PRACTICE PROCEDURAL MANUAL PROJECT (OPTIONAL)

Continue working on your Dental Practice Procedural Manual (see Workbook Chapter 6 for details).
Suggested activities:

- Team meeting
- Review timeline
- Review Group research and writing assignments
- Complete research and writing assignments for this chapter
- Review and revise completed sections of the manual
- Individual journal entries

Jana Rogers

Canyon View Dental Associates
4546 North Avery Way
Canyon View, CA 91783
Telephone (987) 654-3210

Thank you for selecting our dental healthcare team!
We always strive to provide you with the best possible dental care.
To help us meet all your dental healthcare needs, please fill out this form completely.
Please let us know if you have any questions.

Patient Information (CONFIDENTIAL)

Patient # _____

Soc. Sec. # _____

Date _____

Name _____ Birthdate _____ Home Phone _____

Address _____ City _____ State _____ Zip _____

Check Appropriate Box: ☐ Minor ☐ Single ☐ Married ☐ Divorced ☐ Widowed ☐ Separated

Patient's or Parent's Employer _____ Work Phone _____

Business Address _____ City _____ State _____ Zip _____

Spouse or Parent's Name _____ Employer _____ Work Phone _____

If Patient is a Student, Name of School/College _____ City _____ State ____ Zip _____

Whom May We Thank for Referring you? _____

Person to Contact in Case of Emergency _____ Phone _____

Responsible Party

Name of Person Responsible for this Account _____ Relationship to Patient _____

Address _____ Home Phone _____

Driver's License # _____ Birthdate _____ Financial Information _____

Employer _____ Work Phone _____

Is this Person Currently a Patient in our Office? ☐ Yes ☐ No   Cell Phone _____

Email Address _____

Insurance Information

Name of Insured _____ Relationship to Patient _____

Birthdate _____ Social Security # _____ Date Employed _____

Name of Employer _____ Work Phone _____

Address of Employer _____ City _____ State _____ Zip _____

Insurance Company _____ Group # _____ Union or Local # _____

Ins. Co. Address _____ City _____ State ____ Zip _____

How Much is your Deductible? _____ How much have you met? _____ Max. Annual Benefit _____

DO YOU HAVE ANY ADDITIONAL INSURANCE? ☐ Yes ☐ NO   IF YES, COMPLETE THE FOLLOWING

Name of Insured _____ Relationship to Patient _____

Birthdate _____ Social Security # _____ Date Employed _____

Name of Employer _____ Work Phone _____

Address of Employer _____ City _____ State _____ Zip _____

Insurance Company _____ Group # _____ Union or Local # _____

Ins. Co. Address _____ City _____ State ____ Zip _____

How Much is your Deductible? _____ How much have you met? _____ Max. Annual Benefit _____

I attest to the accuracy of the information on this page.

Patient's or guardian's signature _____ Date _____

REGISTRATION

These forms are intended for student use only

154

Jana Rogers

Canyon View Dental Associates
4546 North Avery Way
Canyon View, CA 91783
Telephone (987) 654-3210

Patient's name _____ Date of birth _____

Chief dental complaint		ORAL HYGIENE	☐ EXCELLENT	☐ GOOD	☐ FAIR	☐ POOR
		CALCULUS	☐ NONE	☐ LITTLE	☐ MODERATE	☐ HEAVY
		PLAQUE	☐ NONE	☐ LITTLE	☐ MODERATE	☐ HEAVY
Blood pressure Pulse		GINGIVAL BLEEDING		☐ LOCALIZED	☐ GENERAL	☐ NONE
		PERIO EXAM	☐ YES	☐ NO		

Oral habits

Existing illness/current drugs

Allergies

New patient current restorations and missing teeth

Oral, soft tissue examination

	Description of any problem
Pharynx	
Tonsils	
Soft palate	
Hard palate	
Tongue	
Floor of mouth	
Buccal mucosa	
Lips skin	
Lymph nodes	
Occlusion	

Crown and bridge

Tooth #	Date placed	Condition

TMJ evaluation

Right	☐ Crepitus	☐ Snapping/popping
Left	☐ Crepitus	☐ Snapping/popping
Tenderness to palpation:		
TMJ	☐ Right	☐ Left
Muscles		
Deviation on closing	RMM	LMM
Needa further TMJ evaluation ☐ Yes ☐ No		
If yes, use TMJ evaluation form		

Extractions

Tooth #	Date extracted

Existing Prosthesis

Max.	Date placed:	Condition:
Min.	Date placed:	Condition:

Date _____

CLINICAL EXAMINATION

These forms are intended for student use only

Jana Rogers

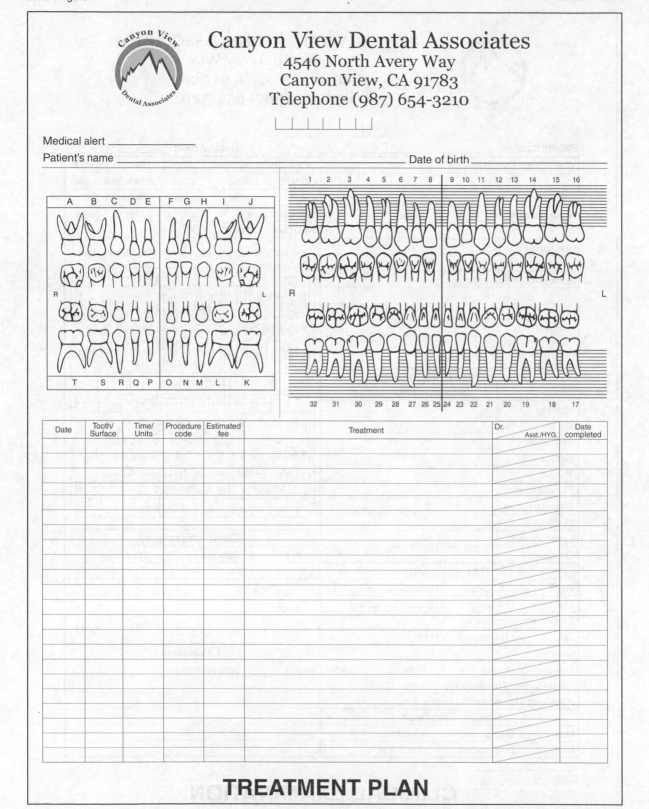

Canyon View Dental Associates
4546 North Avery Way
Canyon View, CA 91783
Telephone (987) 654-3210

Medical alert _____

Patient's name _____ Date of birth _____

Date	Tooth/Surface	Time/Units	Procedure code	Estimated fee	Treatment	Dr. Asst./HYG.	Date completed

TREATMENT PLAN

These forms are intended for student use only

Jana Rogers

Canyon View Dental Associates
4546 North Avery Way
Canyon View, CA 91783
Telephone (987) 654-3210

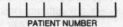

PATIENT NUMBER

PATIENT'S NAME _____
Last   First   Initial

I _____ have had my treatment plan and options explained to me and hereby
authorize this treatment to be performed by Dr. _____

Patient's Signature _____ Date _____
(Parent or Guardian MUST sign if patient is a minor)

I also understand that the cost of this treatment is as follows and that the method of paying for the same
will be:

Total (Partial) estimate of treatment	$	_____
Less:		
Initial Payment	—	_____
Insurance Estimate if Applicable	—	_____
Other _____	—	_____
Balance of Estimate Due	$	_____

Terms: Monthly Payment $ _____ over a _____ month period.

PLEASE CONTACT THE BUSINESS OFFICE IF YOU ARE UNABLE TO MEET YOUR FINANCIAL OBLIGA-
TION

The truth in lending Law enacted in 1969 serves to inform the borrowers and installment purchasers of the true Annual Interest charged on the
amounts financed. This law applies to this office whenever the office extends the courtesy of Installment Payments to our patients, even when no
finance charge is made.

The signature below indicate a mutual understanding of the ESTIMATE for treatment and the acceptable schedule of payment as noted.

Today's Date _____
Signature of Responsible Party

_____
Financial Advisor   Phone Number

Note: THIS IS AN ESTIMATE ONLY, if treatment plan should change please request an amended estimate should it not be offered by our staff.
This estimate is valid for 90 days from the date above IF treatment has not begun within that period. A patient's voluntary termination of treatment
makes this agreement invalid.

FINANCIAL ARRANGEMENTS

These forms are intended for student use only

Alicia Green

Canyon View Dental Associates
4546 North Avery Way
Canyon View, CA 91783
Telephone (987) 654-3210

Thank you for selecting our dental healthcare team!
We always strive to provide you with the best possible dental care.
To help us meet all your dental healthcare needs, please fill out this form completely.
Please let us know if you have any questions.

Patient Information (CONFIDENTIAL)

Patient # _____
Soc. Sec. # _____
Date _____

Name _____ Birthdate _____ Home Phone _____
Address _____ City _____ State _____ Zip _____
Check Appropriate Box: ☐ Minor ☐ Single ☐ Married ☐ Divorced ☐ Widowed ☐ Separated
Patient's or Parent's Employer _____ Work Phone _____
Business Address _____ City _____ State _____ Zip _____
Spouse or Parent's Name _____ Employer _____ Work Phone _____
If Patient is a Student, Name of School/College _____ City _____ State _____ Zip _____
Whom May We Thank for Referring you? _____
Person to Contact in Case of Emergency _____ Phone _____

Responsible Party
Name of Person Responsible for this Account _____ Relationship to Patient _____
Address _____ Home Phone _____
Driver's License # _____ Birthdate _____ Financial Information _____
Employer _____ Work Phone _____
Is this Person Currently a Patient in our Office? ☐ Yes ☐ No   Cell Phone _____
Email Address _____

Insurance Information
Name of Insured _____ Relationship to Patient _____
Birthdate _____ Social Security # _____ Date Employed _____
Name of Employer _____ Work Phone _____
Address of Employer _____ City _____ State _____ Zip _____
Insurance Company _____ Group # _____ Union or Local # _____
Ins. Co. Address _____ City _____ State _____ Zip _____
How Much is your Deductible? _____ How much have you met? _____ Max. Annual Benefit _____

DO YOU HAVE ANY ADDITIONAL INSURANCE? ☐ Yes ☐ NO   IF YES, COMPLETE THE FOLLOWING

Name of Insured _____ Relationship to Patient _____
Birthdate _____ Social Security # _____ Date Employed _____
Name of Employer _____ Work Phone _____
Address of Employer _____ City _____ State _____ Zip _____
Insurance Company _____ Group # _____ Union or Local # _____
Ins. Co. Address _____ City _____ State _____ Zip _____
How Much is your Deductible? _____ How much have you met? _____ Max. Annual Benefit _____

I attest to the accuracy of the information on this page.

Patient's or guardian's signature _____ Date _____

REGISTRATION

These forms are intended for student use only

Alicia Green

Canyon View Dental Associates
4546 North Avery Way
Canyon View, CA 91783
Telephone (987) 654-3210

Referred by_____ How would you rate the condition of your mouth? ☐ Excellent ☐ Good ☐ Fair ☐ Poor
Previous Dentist _____ How long have you been a patient?_____ Months/Years
Date of most recent dental exam _____/_____/_____ Date of most recent x-rays _____/_____/_____
Date of most recent treatment (other than a cleaning) _____/_____/_____
I routinely see my dentist every: ☐ 3 mo. ☐ 4 mo. ☐ 6 mo. ☐ 12 mo. ☐ Not routinely

WHAT IS YOUR IMMEDIATE CONCERN? _____

PLEASE ANSWER YES OR NO TO THE FOLLOWING: YES   NO

PERSONAL HISTORY

		YES	NO
1.	Are you fearful of dental treatment? How fearful, on a scale of 1 (least) to 10 (most) [____]	☐	☐
2.	Have you had an unfavorable dental experience?	☐	☐
3.	Have you ever had complications from past dental treatment?	☐	☐
4.	Have you ever had trouble getting numb or had any reactions to local anesthetic?	☐	☐
5.	Did you ever have braces, orthodontic treatment or had your bite adjusted?	☐	☐
6.	Have you had any teeth removed?	☐	☐

SMILE CHARACTERISTICS

		YES	NO
7.	Is there anything about the appearance of your teeth that you would like to change?	☐	☐
8.	Have you ever whitened (bleached) your teeth?	☐	☐
9.	Have you felt uncomfortable or self conscious about the appearance of your teeth?	☐	☐
10	Have you been disappointed with the appearance of previous dental work?	☐	☐

BITE AND JAW JOINT

		YES	NO
11.	Do you have problems with your jaw joint? (pain, sounds, limited opening, locking, popping)	☐	☐
12.	Do you / would you have any problems chewing gum?	☐	☐
13.	Do you / would you have any problems chewing bagels, baguettes, protein bars, or other hard foods?	☐	☐
14.	Have your teeth changed in the last 5 years, become shorter, thinner or worn?	☐	☐
15.	Are your teeth crowding or developing spaces?	☐	☐
16.	Do you have more than one bite and squeeze to make your teeth fit together?	☐	☐
17.	Do you chew ice, bite your nails, use your teeth to hold objects, or have any other oral habits?	☐	☐
18.	Do you clench your teeth in the daytime or make them sore?	☐	☐
19.	Do you have any problems with sleep or wake up with an awareness of your teeth?	☐	☐
20.	Do you wear or have you ever worn a bite appliance?	☐	☐

TOOTH STRUCTURE

		YES	NO
21.	Have you had any cavities within the past 3 years?	☐	☐
22.	Does the amount of saliva in your mouth seem too little or do you have difficulty swallowing any food?	☐	☐
23.	Do you feel or notice any holes (i.e. pitting, craters) on the biting surface of your teeth?	☐	☐
24.	Are any teeth sensitive to hot, cold, biting, sweets, or avoid brushing any part of your mouth?	☐	☐
25.	Do you have grooves or notches on your teeth near the gum line?	☐	☐
26.	Have you ever broken teeth, chipped teeth, or had a toothache or cracked filling?	☐	☐
27.	Do you get food caught between any teeth?	☐	☐

GUM AND BONE

		YES	NO
28.	Do your gums bleed when brushing or flossing?	☐	☐
29.	Have you ever been treated for gum disease or been told you have lost bone around your teeth?	☐	☐
30.	Have you ever noticed an unpleasant taste or odor in your mouth?	☐	☐
31.	Is there anyone with a history of periodontal disease in your family?	☐	☐
32.	Have you ever experienced gum recession?	☐	☐
33.	Have you ever had any teeth become loose on their own (without an injury), or do you have difficulty eating an apple?	☐	☐
34.	Have you experienced a burning sensation in your mouth?	☐	☐

Patient's Signature _____ Date_____

Doctor's Signature _____ Date_____

DENTAL HISTORY

These forms are intended for student use only

Canyon View Dental Associates
4546 North Avery Way
Canyon View, CA 91783
Telephone (987) 654-3210

MEDICAL HISTORY

Patient Name _____ Nickname _____ Age _____
Name of Physician/and their specialty _____
Most recent physical examination _____ Purpose _____
What is your estimate of your general health? ☐Excellent ☐Good ☐Fair ☐Poor

DO YOU HAVE or HAVE YOU EVER HAD: YES NO

1. hospitalization for illness or injury_____ ☐ ☐
2. an allergic reaction to
   - ☐ aspirin, ibuprofen, acetaminophen, codeine
   - ☐ penicillin
   - ☐ erythromycin
   - ☐ tetracycline
   - ☐ sulpha
   - ☐ local anesthetic
   - ☐ fluoride
   - ☐ metals (nickel, gold, silver, _____)
   - ☐ latex
   - ☐ other _____
3. heart problems, or cardiac stent within the last six months __ ☐ ☐
4. history of infective endocarditis _____ ☐ ☐
5. artificial heart valve, repaired heart defect (PFO) _____ ☐ ☐
6. pacemaker or implantable defibrillator _____ ☐ ☐
7. artificial prosthesis (heart valve or joints) _____ ☐ ☐
8. rheumatic or scarlet fever_____ ☐ ☐
9. high or low blood pressure_____ ☐ ☐
10. a stroke (taking blood thinners) _____ ☐ ☐
11. anemia or other blood disorder _____ ☐ ☐
12. prolonged bleeding due to a slight cut (INR > 3.5) _____ ☐ ☐
13. emphysema, sarcoidosis _____ ☐ ☐
14. tuberculosis _____ ☐ ☐
15. asthma _____ ☐ ☐
16. breathing or sleep problems (i.e. snoring, sinus)_____ ☐ ☐
17. kidney disease _____ ☐ ☐
18. liver disease _____ ☐ ☐
19. jaundice _____ ☐ ☐
20. thyroid, parathyroid disease, or calcium deficiency _____ ☐ ☐
21. hormone deficiency _____ ☐ ☐
22. high cholesterol or taking statin drugs _____ ☐ ☐
23. diabetes (HbA1c = _____) _____ ☐ ☐
24. stomach or duodenal ulcer _____ ☐ ☐
25. digestive disorders (i.e. gastric reflux)_____ ☐ ☐

   YES NO

26. osteoporosis/osteopenia (i.e. taking bisphosphonates) __ ☐ ☐
27. arthritis _____ ☐ ☐
28. glaucoma _____ ☐ ☐
29. contact lenses _____ ☐ ☐
30. head or neck injuries _____ ☐ ☐
31. epilepsy, convulsions (seizures) _____ ☐ ☐
32. neurologic problems (attention deficit disorder) _____ ☐ ☐
33. viral infections and cold sores _____ ☐ ☐
34. any lumps or swelling in the mouth_____ ☐ ☐
35. hives, skin rash, hay fever_____ ☐ ☐
36. venereal disease _____ ☐ ☐
37. hepatitis (type ___) _____ ☐ ☐
38. HIV / AIDS _____ ☐ ☐
39. tumor, abnormal growth_____ ☐ ☐
40. radiation therapy _____ ☐ ☐
41. chemotherapy_____ ☐ ☐
42. emotional problems _____ ☐ ☐
43. psychiatric treatment_____ ☐ ☐
44. antidepressant medication _____ ☐ ☐
45. alcohol / drug dependency _____ ☐ ☐

ARE YOU:

46. presently being treated for any other illness _____ ☐ ☐
47. aware of a change in your general health _____ ☐ ☐
48. taking medication for weight management (i.e. fen-phen) ☐ ☐
49. taking dietary supplements_____ ☐ ☐
50. often exhausted or fatigued _____ ☐ ☐
51. subject to frequent headaches _____ ☐ ☐
52. a smoker or smoked previously _____ ☐ ☐
53. considered a touchy person _____ ☐ ☐
54. often unhappy or depressed _____ ☐ ☐
55. FEMALE - taking birth control pills _____ ☐ ☐
56. FEMALE - pregnant _____ ☐ ☐
57. MALE - prostate disorders _____ ☐ ☐

Describe any current medical treatment, impending surgery, or other treatment that may possibly affect your dental treatment.
_____

List all medications, supplements, and or vitamins taken within the last two years

Drug	Purpose	Drug	Purpose
_____	_____	_____	_____
_____	_____	_____	_____
_____	_____	_____	_____

Ask for an additional sheet if you are taking more than 6 medications

PLEASE ADVISE US IN THE FUTURE OF ANY CHANGE IN YOUR MEDICAL HISTORY OR ANY MEDICATIONS YOU MAY BE TAKING.

Patient's Signature _____ Date _____
Doctor's Signature _____ Date _____

MEDICAL HISTORY

These forms are intended for student use only

Alicia Green

Canyon View Dental Associates
4546 North Avery Way
Canyon View, CA 91783
Telephone (987) 654-3210

Patient's name _____ Date of birth _____

Chief dental complaint		ORAL HYGIENE	☐EXCELLENT	☐GOOD	☐FAIR	☐POOR
		CALCULUS	☐NONE	☐LITTLE	☐MODERATE	☐HEAVY
		PLAQUE	☐NONE	☐LITTLE	☐MODERATE	☐HEAVY
Blood pressure	Pulse	GINGIVAL BLEEDING		☐LOCALIZED	☐GENERAL	☐NONE
		PERIO EXAM	☐YES	☐NO		

Oral habits

Existing illness/current drugs

Allergies

New patient current restorations and missing teeth

Oral, soft tissue examination

	Description of any problem
Pharynx	
Tonsils	
Soft palate	
Hard palate	
Tongue	
Floor of mouth	
Buccal mucosa	
Lips skin	
Lymph nodes	
Occlusion	

Crown and bridge

Tooth #	Date placed	Condition

TMJ evaluation

Right	☐ Crepitus	☐ Snapping/popping
Left	☐ Crepitus	☐ Snapping/popping
Tenderness to palpation:		
TMJ	☐ Right	☐ Left
Muscles		
Deviation on closing	RMM	LMM
Needa further TMJ evaluation	☐ Yes	☐ No
If yes, use TMJ evaluation form		

Extractions

Tooth #	Date extracted

Existing Prosthesis

Max.	Date placed:	Condition:
Min.	Date placed:	Condition:

Date _____

CLINICAL EXAMINATION

These forms are intended for student use only

Canyon View Dental Associates
4546 North Avery Way
Canyon View, CA 91783
Telephone (987) 654-3210

PATIENT'S NAME _____

| Last | First | Initial | Date of Birth |

DATE _____ THERAPIST _____

PROBING – Place probe as close to the contact point as possible, directed along the long axis of the tooth. Take the mesial, mid and distal measurements from the buccal aspect. Repeat for lingual aspect. Record only those measurements over 3mm.

BLEEDING – After probing each quadrant, note whether or not bleeding has occurred. Indicate the bleeding area by circling the pocket in red.

MOBILITY – Move each tooth between two instrument handles in a bucco-lingual direction and attempt to depress each tooth in its socket. Grade each tooth accordingly: 0 - Movement of less than 0.5mm; 1 - 0.5mm to 1.0mm; 2 - 1.0mm to 2.0mm; 3 - Movement of more that 2.0mm or depressible.

FURCATION – Probe from the buccal and lingual. Record accordingly: 0 - Normal; 1 - Slight; 2 - Moderate; 3 - Through and through.

RECESSION – Measure the exposed surface from the cemental enamel junction (CEJ) to the gingival crest. Enter the distance in millimeters (mm).

R (upper chart, teeth 1–16) **L**

Date/Therapist | Tooth 1 2 3 4 5 6 7 8 | 9 10 11 12 13 14 15 16 (columns D M for each tooth)
Rows: Pocket Depth B/L, Mobility, Furcation, Recession (three date blocks)

R (lower chart, teeth 32–17) **L**

Date/Therapist | Tooth 32 31 30 29 28 27 26 25 | 24 23 22 21 20 19 18 17
Rows: Pocket Depth B/L, Mobility, Furcation, Recession (three date blocks)

| Enter highest POCKET DEPTH score in appropriate box | ☐ Any pocket depth reading from 3 to 5mm, read below | ☐ Any pocket depth reading over 5mm, read below |
| Enter highest MOBILITY SCORE in appropriate box | ☐ Any mobility of 1, read below | ☐ Any mobility of 2 or 3, read below |

BLEEDING ☐ When any bleeding upon probing is noted, read below

INSTRUMENTS FOR TREATMENT SELECTION
Locate square containing score farthest to the right and follow treatment, listed below.

☐ Explanation of periodontal disease.

Gingivitis
A. Hygienist Treatment
1. Oral Hygiene Instruction
2. Prophylaxis

Moderate Periodontitis
OPTION 1
A. Dentist or Hygienist Treatment
1. Oral Hygiene Instruction
2. Periodontal Root Planing
3. Occlusal Analysis
4. Maintenance Recall
OPTION 2
B. Referral to Periodontist

Advanced Periodontitis
OPTION 1
A. Referral to Periodontist
OPTION 2
B. Dentist Treatment
1. Oral Hygiene Instruction
2. Periodontal Root Planing
3. Occlusal Analysis
4. Periodontal Surgery
5. Splinting
6. Maintenance Recall

PERIODONTAL SCREENING EXAMINATION

These forms are intended for student use only

Chapter **Appendix: Patient Paperwork**

Alicia Green

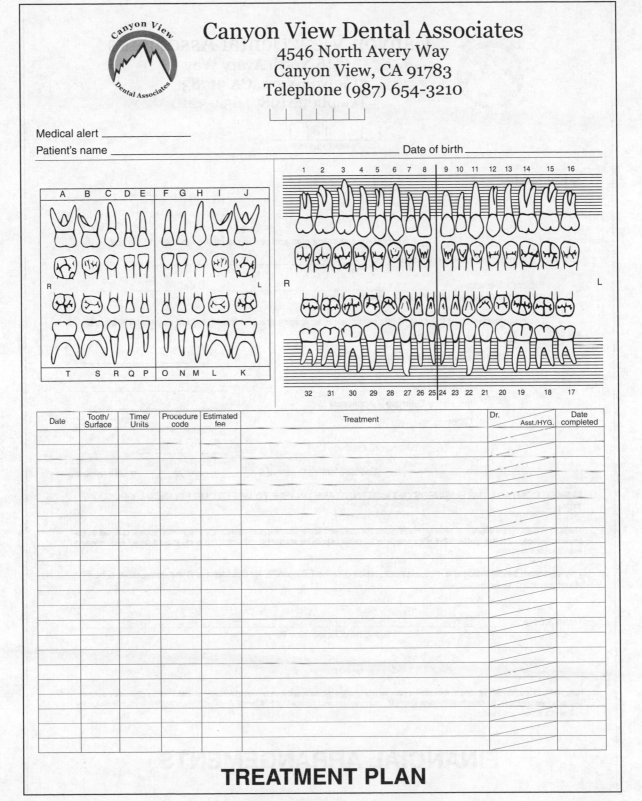

Canyon View Dental Associates
4546 North Avery Way
Canyon View, CA 91783
Telephone (987) 654-3210

Medical alert _____
Patient's name _____ Date of birth _____

Date	Tooth/ Surface	Time/ Units	Procedure code	Estimated fee	Treatment	Dr. Asst./HYG.	Date completed

TREATMENT PLAN

These forms are intended for student use only

Alicia Green

Canyon View Dental Associates
4546 North Avery Way
Canyon View, CA 91783
Telephone (987) 654-3210

PATIENT NUMBER

PATIENT'S NAME _____

                                   Last   First   Initial

I _____ have had my treatment plan and options explained to me and hereby authorize this treatment to be performed by Dr. _____

Patient's Signature _____ Date _____
(Parent or Guardian MUST sign if patient is a minor)

I also understand that the cost of this treatment is as follows and that the method of paying for the same will be:

Total (Partial) estimate of treatment	$_____
Less:	
Initial Payment	—_____
Insurance Estimate if Applicable	—_____
Other _____	—_____
Balance of Estimate Due	$_____

Terms: Monthly Payment $ _____ over a _____ month period.

PLEASE CONTACT THE BUSINESS OFFICE IF YOU ARE UNABLE TO MEET YOUR FINANCIAL OBLIGATION

The truth in lending Law enacted in 1969 serves to inform the borrowers and installment purchasers of the true Annual Interest charged on the amounts financed. This law applies to this office whenever the office extends the courtesy of Installment Payments to our patients, even when no finance charge is made.

The signature below indicate a mutual understanding of the ESTIMATE for treatment and the acceptable schedule of payment as noted.

Today's Date _____
                                        Signature of Responsible Party

_____
                    Financial Advisor   Phone Number

Note: THIS IS AN ESTIMATE ONLY, if treatment plan should change please request an amended estimate should it not be offered by our staff. This estimate is valid for 90 days from the date above IF treatment has not begun within that period. A patient's voluntary termination of treatment makes this agreement invalid.

FINANCIAL ARRANGEMENTS

These forms are intended for student use only

Holly Barry

Canyon View Dental Associates
4546 North Avery Way
Canyon View, CA 91783
Telephone (987) 654-3210

Thank you for selecting our dental healthcare team!
We always strive to provide you with the best possible dental care.
To help us meet all your dental healthcare needs, please fill out this form completely.
Please let us know if you have any questions.

Patient Information (CONFIDENTIAL)

Patient # _____
Soc. Sec. # _____
Date _____

Name _____ Birthdate _____ Home Phone _____

Address _____ City _____ State _____ Zip _____

Check Appropriate Box: ☐ Minor ☐ Single ☐ Married ☐ Divorced ☐ Widowed ☐ Separated

Patient's or Parent's Employer _____ Work Phone _____

Business Address _____ City _____ State _____ Zip _____

Spouse or Parent's Name _____ Employer_____ Work Phone_____

If Patient is a Student, Name of School/College _____ City_____ State _____ Zip _____

Whom May We Thank for Referring you? _____

Person to Contact in Case of Emergency _____ Phone _____

Responsible Party

Name of Person Responsible for this Account _____ Relationship to Patient _____

Address _____ Home Phone_____

Driver's License # _____ Birthdate _____ Financial Information _____

Employer_____ Work Phone _____

Is this Person Currently a Patient in our Office? ☐ Yes ☐ No

Cell Phone _____
Email Address _____

Insurance Information

Name of Insured _____ Relationship to Patient _____

Birthdate_____ Social Security # _____ Date Employed _____

Name of Employer _____ Work Phone _____

Address of Employer _____ City _____ State _____ Zip _____

Insurance Company_____ Group # _____ Union or Local # _____

Ins. Co. Address _____ City _____ State _____ Zip _____

How Much is your Deductible? _____ How much have you met? _____ Max. Annual Benefit _____

DO YOU HAVE ANY ADDITIONAL INSURANCE? ☐ Yes ☐ N0   IF YES, COMPLETE THE FOLLOWING

Name of Insured _____ Relationship to Patient _____

Birthdate _____ Social Security #_____ Date Employed _____

Name of Employer_____ Work Phone _____

Address of Employer _____ City_____ State _____ Zip _____

Insurance Company_____ Group #_____ Union or Local # _____

Ins. Co. Address _____ City_____ State _____ Zip _____

How Much is your Deductible? _____ How much have you met? _____ Max. Annual Benefit _____

I attest to the accuracy of the information on this page.

Patient's or guardian's signature _____ Date _____

REGISTRATION

These forms are intended for student use only

165

Canyon View Dental Associates

4546 North Avery Way
Canyon View, CA 91783
Telephone (987) 654-3210

Patient's name _____   Date of birth _____

Chief dental complaint			ORAL HYGIENE	☐ EXCELLENT	☐ GOOD	☐ FAIR	☐ POOR

		CALCULUS	☐ NONE	☐ LITTLE	☐ MODERATE	☐ HEAVY

		PLAQUE	☐ NONE	☐ LITTLE	☐ MODERATE	☐ HEAVY

Blood pressure Pulse		GINGIVAL BLEEDING	☐ LOCALIZED	☐ GENERAL	☐ NONE

		PERIO EXAM	☐ YES	☐ NO

Oral habits

Existing illness/current drugs

Allergies

Oral, soft tissue examination

New patient current restorations and missing teeth

	Description of any problem
Pharynx	
Tonsils	
Soft palate	
Hard palate	
Tongue	
Floor of mouth	
Buccal mucosa	
Lips skin	
Lymph nodes	
Occlusion	

Crown and bridge

Tooth #	Date placed	Condition

TMJ evaluation

Right	☐ Crepitus	☐ Snapping/popping
Left	☐ Crepitus	☐ Snapping/popping
Tenderness to palpation:		
TMJ	☐ Right	☐ Left
Muscles		
Deviation on closing	RMM	LMM
Needa further TMJ evaluation	☐ Yes	☐ No
If yes, use TMJ evaluation form		

Extractions

Tooth #	Date extracted

Existing Prosthesis

Max.	Date placed:	Condition:
Min.	Date placed:	Condition:

_____
Date

CLINICAL EXAMINATION

These forms are intended for student use only

Holly Barry

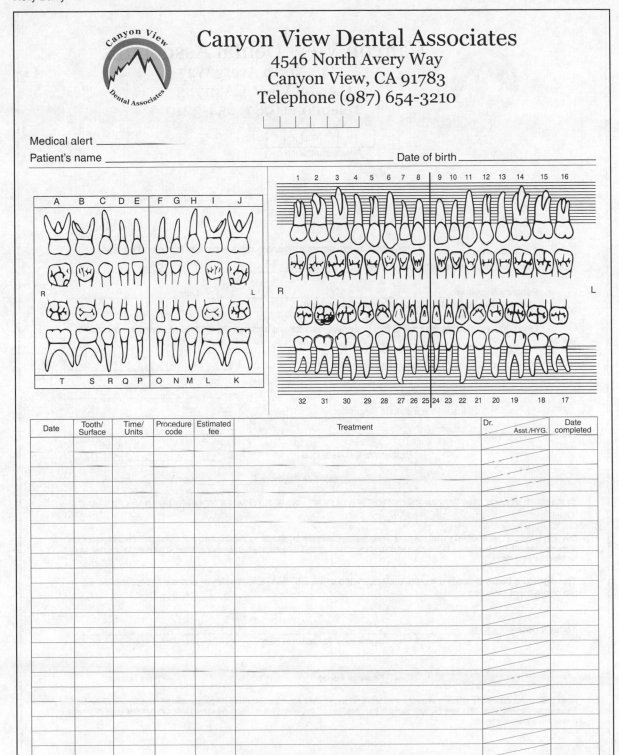

Canyon View Dental Associates
4546 North Avery Way
Canyon View, CA 91783
Telephone (987) 654-3210

Medical alert _____

Patient's name _____ Date of birth _____

Date	Tooth/ Surface	Time/ Units	Procedure code	Estimated fee	Treatment	Dr. Asst./HYG.	Date completed

TREATMENT PLAN

These forms are intended for student use only

Canyon View Dental Associates
4546 North Avery Way
Canyon View, CA 91783
Telephone (987) 654-3210

PATIENT NUMBER

PATIENT'S NAME _____
Last   First   Initial

I _____ have had my treatment plan and options explained to me and hereby authorize this treatment to be performed by Dr. _____

Patient's Signature _____ Date _____
  (Parent or Guardian MUST sign if patient is a minor)

I also understand that the cost of this treatment is as follows and that the method of paying for the same will be:

Total (Partial) estimate of treatment	$ _____
Less:	
Initial Payment	− _____
Insurance Estimate if Applicable	− _____
Other _____	− _____
Balance of Estimate Due	$ _____

Terms: Monthly Payment $ _____ over a _____ month period.

PLEASE CONTACT THE BUSINESS OFFICE IF YOU ARE UNABLE TO MEET YOUR FINANCIAL OBLIGATION

The truth in lending Law enacted in 1969 serves to inform the borrowers and installment purchasers of the true Annual Interest charged on the amounts financed. This law applies to this office whenever the office extends the courtesy of Installment Payments to our patients, even when no finance charge is made.

The signature below indicate a mutual understanding of the ESTIMATE for treatment and the acceptable schedule of payment as noted.

Today's Date _____
        Signature of Responsible Party

_____
Financial Advisor   Phone Number

Note: THIS IS AN ESTIMATE ONLY, if treatment plan should change please request an amended estimate should it not be offered by our staff. This estimate is valid for 90 days from the date above IF treatment has not begun within that period. A patient's voluntary termination of treatment makes this agreement invalid.

FINANCIAL ARRANGEMENTS

These forms are intended for student use only

Lynn Bacca

Canyon View Dental Associates
4546 North Avery Way
Canyon View, CA 91783
Telephone (987) 654-3210

Thank you for selecting our dental healthcare team!
We always strive to provide you with the best possible dental care.
To help us meet all your dental healthcare needs, please fill out this form completely.
Please let us know if you have any questions.

Patient Information (CONFIDENTIAL)

Patient # _____

Soc. Sec. # _____

Date _____

Name _____ Birthdate _____ Home Phone _____

Address _____ City _____ State _____ Zip _____

Check Appropriate Box: ☐ Minor ☐ Single ☐ Married ☐ Divorced ☐ Widowed ☐ Separated

Patient's or Parent's Employer _____ Work Phone _____

Business Address _____ City _____ State _____ Zip _____

Spouse or Parent's Name _____ Employer_____ Work Phone _____

If Patient is a Student, Name of School/College _____ City _____ State _____ Zip _____

Whom May We Thank for Referring you? _____

Person to Contact in Case of Emergency _____ Phone _____

Responsible Party

Name of Person Responsible for this Account _____ Relationship to Patient _____

Address _____ Home Phone _____

Driver's License # _____ Birthdate _____ Financial Information _____

Employer_____ Work Phone _____

Is this Person Currently a Patient in our Office? ☐ Yes ☐ No   Cell Phone _____

Email Address _____

Insurance Information

Name of Insured_____ Relationship to Patient _____

Birthdate_____ Social Security #_____ Date Employed _____

Name of Employer _____ Work Phone _____

Address of Employer _____ City _____ State _____ Zip _____

Insurance Company_____ Group # _____ Union or Local # _____

Ins. Co. Address _____ City _____ State _____ Zip _____

How Much is your Deductible? _____ How much have you met? _____ Max. Annual Benefit _____

DO YOU HAVE ANY ADDITIONAL INSURANCE? ☐ Yes ☐ NO   IF YES, COMPLETE THE FOLLOWING

Name of Insured _____ Relationship to Patient _____

Birthdate _____ Social Security #_____ Date Employed _____

Name of Employer_____ Work Phone _____

Address of Employer _____ City_____ State _____ Zip _____

Insurance Company_____ Group #_____ Union or Local #_____

Ins. Co. Address _____ City_____ State _____ Zip _____

How Much is your Deductible? _____ How much have you met? _____ Max. Annual Benefit _____

I attest to the accuracy of the information on this page.

Patient's or guardian's signature _____ Date _____

REGISTRATION

These forms are intended for student use only

Chapter   **Appendix: Patient Paperwork**

Canyon View Dental Associates
4546 North Avery Way
Canyon View, CA 91783
Telephone (987) 654-3210

Patient's name _____ Date of birth _____

Chief dental complaint	ORAL HYGIENE	☐EXCELLENT	☐GOOD	☐FAIR	☐POOR
	CALCULUS	☐NONE	☐LITTLE	☐MODERATE	☐HEAVY
	PLAQUE	☐NONE	☐LITTLE	☐MODERATE	☐HEAVY
Blood pressure Pulse	GINGIVAL BLEEDING		☐LOCALIZED	☐GENERAL	☐NONE
	PERIO EXAM	☐YES	☐NO		

Oral habits

Existing illness/current drugs

Allergies

New patient current restorations and missing teeth

[Tooth chart]

Oral, soft tissue examination

	Description of any problem
Pharynx	
Tonsils	
Soft palate	
Hard palate	
Tongue	
Floor of mouth	
Buccal mucosa	
Lips skin	
Lymph nodes	
Occlusion	

Crown and bridge

Tooth #	Date placed	Condition

TMJ evaluation

Right	☐ Crepitus	☐ Snapping/popping
Left	☐ Crepitus	☐ Snapping/popping
Tenderness to palpation:		
TMJ	☐ Right	☐ Left
Muscles		
Deviation on closing RMM LMM		
Needa further TMJ evaluation ☐ Yes ☐ No		
If yes, use TMJ evaluation form		

Extractions

Tooth #	Date extracted

Existing Prosthesis

Max.	Date placed:	Condition:
Min.	Date placed:	Condition:

Date _____

CLINICAL EXAMINATION

These forms are intended for student use only

Lynn Bacca

Canyon View Dental Associates
4546 North Avery Way
Canyon View, CA 91783
Telephone (987) 654-3210

Medical alert _____

Patient's name _____ Date of birth _____

Date	Tooth/ Surface	Time/ Units	Procedure code	Estimated fee	Treatment	Dr. Asst./HYG.	Date completed

TREATMENT PLAN

These forms are intended for student use only

Canyon View Dental Associates

4546 North Avery Way
Canyon View, CA 91783
Telephone (987) 654-3210

⌊ | | | | | ⌋
PATIENT NUMBER

PATIENT'S NAME _____

Last   First   Initial

I _____ have had my treatment plan and options explained to me and hereby

authorize this treatment to be performed by Dr. _____

Patient's Signature _____ Date_____
(Parent or Guardian MUST sign if patient is a minor)

I also understand that the cost of this treatment is as follows and that the method of paying for the same
will be:

Total (Partial) estimate of treatment	$_____
Less:	
Initial Payment	—_____
Insurance Estimate if Applicable	—_____
Other _____	—_____
Balance of Estimate Due	$_____

Terms: Monthly Payment $_____ over a _____ month period.

PLEASE CONTACT THE BUSINESS OFFICE IF YOU ARE UNABLE TO MEET YOUR FINANCIAL OBLIGA-
TION

The truth in lending Law enacted in 1969 serves to inform the borrowers and installment purchasers of the true Annual Interest charged on the
amounts financed. This law applies to this office whenever the office extends the courtesy of Installment Payments to our patients, even when no
finance charge is made.

The signature below indicate a mutual understanding of the ESTIMATE for treatment and the acceptable schedule of payment as noted.

Today's Date _____

Signature of Responsible Party

_____

Financial Advisor   Phone Number

Note: THIS IS AN ESTIMATE ONLY, if treatment plan should change please request an amended estimate should it not be offered by our staff.
This estimate is valid for 90 days from the date above IF treatment has not begun within that period. A patient's voluntary termination of treatment
makes this agreement invalid.

FINANCIAL ARRANGEMENTS

These forms are intended for student use only